THE NURSE
IN THE
WORKPLACE

A NURSES NOTES

To Dr Flores

MARCO A. GONZALEZ,
NURSE EDUCATOR

Thank You For Your Support

authorHOUSE®

AuthorHouse™
1663 Liberty Drive
Bloomington, IN 47403
www.authorhouse.com
Phone: 1 (800) 839-8640

Published by AuthorHouse   05/26/2020

ISBN: 978-1-7283-6083-6 (sc)
ISBN: 978-1-7283-6082-9 (hc)
ISBN: 978-1-7283-6081-2 (e)

Library of Congress Control Number: 2020908417

Print information available on the last page.

Scripture quotations marked KJV are from the Holy Bible, King James Version
(Authorized Version). First published in 1611. Quoted from the KJV Classic
Reference Bible, Copyright © 1983 by The Zondervan Corporation.

This book is printed on acid-free paper.

Dedicated to my Mother,
A Prayer Warrior, for her faith in me.

Also to my children Miriam, Marco Taino and Kris

Special thanks to Irma Beniquez, R.N.
who advised me professionally.

Also thanks to Sarah B. Breire, R.N.,
F.N.P who inspired this book.

For all Licensed Practical Nurses who have
dedicated themselves to This Art of Nursing.

To all the nurses, on every level and
specialty that inspired this work.

A Special Thank You Rev. Pastor Jim Cymbala
of The Brooklyn Tabernacle.

CONTENTS

Preface xi
About the Author xiii

1   The Licensed Practical Nurse 1
2   Education 24
3   Choosing An Area Of Practice 39
4   Professional Enhancements 50
5   Diversity 62
6   Flexibility 71
7   Taking Charge 86
8   Independent Practice 105
9   Nurse Contractor/Vender 121
10 Medical-Legal Aspects 130

There is no room for bias

In the practice of nursing

We may not like what we see.

We may not like what we hear ......

However, goodness will prevail

Through it all

Marco A. Gonzalez

PREFACE

A NURSES NOTES IS about the journey of a male nurse that has entered the profession of nursing and the realms of healthcare. A journey that hopes to enlighten and motivate anyone, that desires to be a part of the greatest and vast of the nursing and healthcare professions. There are introductions to various areas of healthcare and inter-related organizations and corporate entities.

First and Foremost I am grateful to The Lord for taking me through this journey. A very special thanks, to all who have supported me in this journey. To name a few, Eusebio Beniquez, who encouraged me by faith to begin this journey. Shirley Bloomfield, R.N, D.N.S. who opened the first door. Ruth Goldberg RN, A.D.N. who pushed me not to look back. Joseph Fiorentino, R.N., MSN. who introduce me to the halls of critical care. Harvey Goldberg, M.D. who demonstrated that I could do this, Michael Becker, Esq, Lester Kravitz Esq. who supported me through so much including 9-11-01. Rosalie Richardson who provided every which way I would go. Captain Harris MD, USN Medical Corps, who believed in me to lead in ways that saved so many. Dr. Cochran for his guidance in academia.

For the most part are there are anecdotes of experiences that are hoped to encourage and open an understanding of what it is like to serve your fellow man without reservations. To develop an understanding of what nurses in the world may go through while providing unselfish love to humanity. Not only to humanity but also to wildlife and the environment in which we all live.

ABOUT THE AUTHOR

MARCO A. GONZALEZ entered the practical nursing field in 1973 and graduated in 1974. Since then he has diversified the role of he L.P.N.. He attended college on independent study levels, which include electives in psychology, anatomy and physiology as well as communications and cultural studies. He also did a stint in legal studies at The New York State Trial Lawyers Association School in New York City. He then earned professional teaching licenses in New York State by The University of The State of New York as a private school teacher in the areas of electrocardiography, phlebotomy, medical assistants, medical office management, and certified nurses assistant theory also, becoming a Certified Allied Health Instructor by the American Association of Medical Technologists.

In 1988 he joined the United States Naval Reserve as a Petty Officer and taught various subjects in military medicine to independent duty corpsman for field operations, ships and submarine squadrons. In 1990 he was awarded the National Defense Medal and the New York State Medal for his efforts in the Persian Gulf Crisis after being mobilized for active duty by President George Bush and serving in Operation Desert Storm/Desert Shield. He served as an instructor for independent duty corpsman: as a Leading Petty Officer, supporting submarine squadrons, sea and shore teams.

These experiences came together on September 11, 2001 serving the public and his country between Bellevue Hospital and Ground Zero World Trade Center New York City disaster. He has brought forty-five years of multilevel health care experience to the work place.

Irma I. G Beniquez, R. N.

CHAPTER ONE

THE LICENSED PRACTICAL NURSE

S INCE THE INCEPTION of the licensed practical nurse, (Mid 1800 Crimea War in London and 1896 Spanish American War nursing health effort) Vancouver Island University of Practical Nursing Guide, n. d.) Implemented, also, by The United States Army Nurse Corps and The United States Navy Nurse Corps in 1901 and made permanent in 1908, as a helpful and permanent establishment which improved and continues to improve the education of professional licensed practical nurses to date. Initially trained and educated by The American Red Cross, the United States Army Nurse Corps and the United States Navy Nurse Corps in WWI. This practice of nursing endures. When there were no specially battlefield-trained persons, military, civilian or otherwise, select civilians were educated and specifically trained to rescue and tend to the wounded soldiers and sailors in the theater of war and crisis.

The licensed practical nurse is a dedicated integral member of the health care delivery system, the patient/client being first and foremost and providing the highest and outstanding level of healthcare. Endeavoring, learning and applying theory to the practice of professional licensed practical nursing; develops a well-rounded foundation for delivering professional nursing services. Becoming familiar with the patient/client, therefore, understanding the patient/clients needs, will align the professionally licensed nurse for the performance of exceptional care. By understanding the professional medical and nursing guidelines as well as the professional medical protocols within the practical nursing scope of practice and applying nursing theory, develops a well-founded structure for the delivery of professional nursing services. In this professional practice of practical nursing, demands may vary, from client to client. Be it one client/patient or many client/patients including organizations on a continuum. We learn at a one at a time pace but practice on a multi-level continuum. A continuum may be on a single diagnostic or even on a multi-diagnostic level. The latter usually being the practice.

By professionally distinguishing who the clients are and what their needs may be, will define and produce the pathways and vehicle by which the performance of professional nursing may be experienced. Developing a fundamental and comprehensive understanding of age specific groups, the specific and relative diagnosis, as well as, age specific guidelines and protocols, may provide a clear comprehension on the role of the professionally licensed nurse; whether it is prenatal services for the childbearing mother, the neonate, born new to the world, a child with developing milestones or an adult in need of nursing care. The colors on the canvas for this art of professional nursing will provide the necessary knowledge with scope of practice. Continually being aware and prepared to meet the needs of the client/patient will result in a well-performed professional nursing service.

Continually preparing and endeavoring to provide professional, consistent and outstanding quality nursing care, to all in need of professional nursing services, will attain outstanding quality outcomes. Whereas, the role of the professional licensed practical nurse maintains its place, in the realms of professional healthcare. There are a multitude of general, clinical and specialty areas in which the professionally licensed nurse may provide professional nursing services. Comprehensive communication with the recipient of healthcare by the professionally licensed nurse is essential. The preparations required for professional performance at the clinical setting will vary. From general medical and nursing professional practice to specialty medical and nursing practices. The professional communications, respectful of the patient and their families, with the clear understanding of the HIPPA laws, will prevent unnecessary insult or litigation. That is, respectful of the Health Information Portability Privacy Act (HIPPA), being professionally mindful, to protect the patient/client rights to care on such healthcare continuum.

Practical nursing school is not a walk in the park. It would appear, to the pre-nursing students, that becoming a professional practical nurse is like becoming a professional registered nurse, but not really. Becoming a professional licensed practical nurse requires being ready, for a continuous and consistent one-year course, with a well-planned effort. Colleges may provide practical nursing education, preparation and training, in continual semesters. Whereby, and inclusively, scheduling collegiate elective courses. Private schools, such as the one that I graduated from, on the other hand, provide continuous classroom theory and clinical practice.

Along with the education, training and preparations for practical nursing are professional foundations of medical and surgical didactics, alternating with clinical practice and rotations. These clinical and classroom rotations are for the introductions to the general medical and surgical clinical settings, as well as the respective specialties for professional medical and nursing practice.

Long days and studious hours will seem like an eternity. There will be times when your eyes just want to give up and close. There will be times when your mind may feel like it can't find headspace for so much theory. That is when the candidate for professional nursing will be experiencing professional growing pains. By diligently studying, the mind will be etching new theory and facts of life for future implementation. Like, performing exercises at the gymnasium, creating and forming new mental and muscle memory. Time management and prioritizing personal obligations and responsibilities will be the saving grace, for successfully challenging and completing the professional courses. This may take some getting used to. Since the time is actually short, it will be well worth preparing for. After all, the rewards in becoming a professionally licensed nurse will, undoubtedly, out weigh what would not happen if one did not, at least, explore all the possibilities.

Every profession has its own jargon language and scope of practice. Therefore, becoming a professional nurse will enhance your life. Going forward, it will also be the best thing anyone can do. The commitments made will bring a well developed and respected point of professional actualization, and noted. Mankind will be receptive to the tender loving care (TLC) provided to those in need of the professionalism and empathy it takes to deliver such care.

Things that are primary are usually practical. Such as preventive healthcare and follow up implementations. This may range from counseling, applications of immunizations, as well as, medical and or post surgical treatments and procedures. Therefore, the practicality of nursing is essentially hands on. Professionally implementing and skillfully evaluating the practical nursing services throughout the nursing process of nursing care performed. This, also, may take some getting used to. Especially, by starting each day early, planning ahead and trying not to fall short of ones' own obligations and responsibilities. Being attentive to what matters in your day; ones' family, friends, significant others and the things that give great meaning to the reasons that one has chosen to become an integral part of peoples lives.

Long days and hours will seem like an eternity. Schools of practical nursing are not like any other schools. The courses are intense and the practicum is like an emersion. All of the primary phases of healthcare are addressed. Medical nursing which prepares the practical nursing student, in developing primary foundations for delivering nursing care to the patient/client and recording the results of such performed care on a continuum. This continuum will involve an array of medical and nursing professionals, as well as, non-medical or nursing professionals. The first line of professionals will be your fellow professional licensed practical nurses. With the primary nursing orders prescribed by the clients/patients licensed medical doctors. Be it the primary medical doctor and or the referred medical specialist or specialists. Prescribed nursing care may be delegated to the professional licensed practical nurse by the professional registered nurse (R.N.). There are various levels of delegating registered nurses. There is the charge nurse, that is, the nurse receiving the medical doctors orders of the specifics for providing nursing care. There are, also, Nurse Practitioners, Clinical Nurse Specialists and the Physicians Assistant who specialize in the various clinical areas of healthcare.

The primary and practical instructional phases of practical nursing are essential for practicing as a licensed practical nurse. These areas are Medical-Surgical (Med-Surg), Geriatrics (Eldercare), Pediatrics (Peds), Maternal and childcare, which from prenatal antepartum, post partum and care for the newborn and Psychiatric (Mental Health), clinical and community mental health provisions. Community based care are also taught, for a well-rounded understanding of the patients needs. That is, emotional supportiveness, as well as family and social aspects. Specifically, for a focused attention on patient history and data acquisition. Such data may include, but not limited to, psychosocial, medical and surgical past history in relation to family and environmental components.

Surgical nursing instruction orients the practical nursing student to methods and procedures that produce positive results and healing with surgical interventions. This combination of medical-surgical nursing prepares the practical nursing student to professionally deliver bedside and clinical nursing which meet the needs of the patient/client. Thereby placing an emphasis on meeting the healing needs of the patient/client and the family support systems. This will bring the client to understanding their nursing care and, hopefully, that of being independent and the outcomes. Whereby, always encouraging follow up care, health management and maintenance of their health needs.

Geriatric nursing prepares the practical nursing student with foundations in understanding human growth and development in the areas of the aging process, especially the sensitivities and the fragilities of the aged. Especially, how best to provide nursing care of the elderly, infirm and disabled. Protecting the rights of the elderly and infirmed to be understood and respected in their most fragile times. Nurturing the client strengths and strengthening their weaknesses is paramount. Keeping in mind that communication is key.

This fundamental aspect of the aging process will enlighten the practical nursing student in understanding the strengths and abilities of those who built our nation and their contributions to the workplace and the future that was created for mankind. A multicultural and multifaceted population of persons from all over the world including their customs and traditions carried on from generation to generation, respectfully. It is not to say that the practical nurse cannot learn and develop experiences from children, but as we were all once a child we will hopefully be some of the greatest contributors to mankind, by the caring that the licensed practical nurse will bring.

Pediatric nursing instruction prepares the practical nursing student with an understanding of the growth and development milestones of the child development process. This supportive instruction further prepares the practical nurse in delivering client/patient care at the bedside and in a family clinical setting. Pediatric nursing for inpatient and outpatient services will be based on age specific milestones. For example, encouraging the child to participate in their care. Is the child responding to their base line of natural growth and development processes? While evaluating a child's response to care, the practical nurse can also evaluate whether the parenting aspects are being met for the child's growth and development. Immunization schedules and clinical follow up by the parents and caregivers are essential in child healthcare management. Health education relevant to child safety and prevention of illness can be monitored at the clinical level. Understanding the role of the practical nurse in child protective matters. Immunization counseling as well as psychosocial communication tools for gauging age specific milestones and impediments.

Maternal and childcare foundations will provide skills and applications in ante-partum, partum and post- partum nursing care, as well as, parental observational reporting to nursing superiors. Thereby, easing the pains and difficulties of labor and delivery in hospitals and clinics where such services are provided. Counseling the mother through the pre and post natal processes, thereby, facilitating what needs to be done for their infants including all care givers involved in the child rearing and health management process.

How awe-inspiring it is to experience and witness the birth of a child, the wonder of the union of mother and child; the aspirations of parents enjoying their blessings and integration of their children in the world. The practical nursing student will be awed at this primary foundation in maternal and child development. From birth to young adulthood, the phases and milestones will give light to the practical nursing student, when handling peer and community pressure of the growing child. The maturation process will also be introduced with biopsychosocial didactics.

Education in the foundations of psychiatric nursing, for developing an understanding of the emotionally imbalanced patient/client brings a clear vision of the whole person. This is where the reporting of observations of patient/client behaviors, which become paramount in establishing a baseline of mental health. The psychosocial foundations will apply to all phases of educating the professionally licensed nurse, in so much as trauma and illness that will affect emotional stability. The environments and triggers that affect persons with emotional imbalances and the professional licensed nursing care that brings the person with emotional imbalances to a balanced and healthy state of mind.

This integration of classroom and clinical learning experiences will prepare the practical nursing student and be the root tools from which to draw from, tools that will last a lifetime, tools that can and will be enhanced and polished as their service to mankind forges on. If the professionally licensed nurse wore a tool belt at work, it would be too heavy to carry. Therefore, these tools are carried in the heart of each and every professionally licensed nurse. This belt bears the stamp of faith and courage of what it takes to care for persons in need of the empathy and understanding of their infirmity.

Student instruction and supervision bring new awareness to the art of practical nursing. Taken by the hand through the halls of health, and learning, and on the walls of healthcare facilities, will enlighten the practical nursing student in the development of professionalism; working tirelessly through each and every shift, tour of duty and assignments. The desire to soar into the horizons of healthcare will require a further nurturing and willingness to explore and expand the role of the professional licensed practical nurse. Leaps and bounds are only impeded by a lack of desire to succeed.

Where is the professional licensed practical nurse today and where will the professional licensed practical nurse be tomorrow is a current question for the future of the practical nurse. This question is answered through the time and endeavors broadening the horizons of the professionally licensed nurse. It may not lead to narrowing the path of the practical nurse, but may broaden the practices of the professionally licensed nurse. Becoming a professional licensed practical nurse can a stepping-stone or even a cornerstone for future endeavors in nursing and healthcare. The stepping-stones will expand the practices of the licensed practical nurse in future roles and responsibilities. The corner stone will be the strength and the mark going onward and upwards.

In the chapters ahead, there will be shared experiences of the expanded roles of the professionally licensed nurse. The cornerstone will produce the signature statement of the strengths that the professionally licensed nurses' integrity affirms in the fields of nursing and healthcare. The notes and anecdotes of this work are not only to produce stepping-stones; but also, to produce a cornerstone for each and every licensed practical nurse, well founded in the pursuit of healthcare and the well being of mankind and its proponents.

Having gone through the preliminaries and preparations, for becoming a professionally licensed nurse, can bring oneself through the great halls of healthcare and the experiences that will follow. To contribute selflessly for the betterment of mankind is an honor that will be expressed tenfold in time. (One step at a time) Great results can be accomplished with a team effort and a common goal. Faithfully discharging the professional performance and responsibilities for the betterment of mankind.

Presenting oneself professionally, in and out of the work place, will project a professional demeanor for the recipient of professionally licensed nursing services. Becoming a professionally licensed nurse is the same as becoming a new book, be it soft bound or hard bound, the impression given will project how well prepared the professionally licensed nurse is to provide, protect and pursue the positive outcomes for the patient/client. The pages will be read inevitably. The interpretations will be expressed and the words will be delivered professionally. Are you ready is the question that will be answered in the pages of each book? You are the Book.

Always well-groomed and polished, presenting of oneself in a respectable manner and appearance will put a glow on the recipient in your practice. A pleasant voice with clear tone, volume, poise as well as diction will bring a clear response from all persons who you interface with. Therefore, building on the elocutions of professional vocabulary and the appropriate usages from medical ease and nursing ease to provide as clear an understanding as needed, can alleviate misunderstandings and misattributions of professionally licensed nursing practices.

We all have many responsibilities and obligations, which need tending to. Beginning with our family and our community, the practical nurse will learn to implement time and stress management techniques. This will better prepare the licensed nurse in developing a balance between home and the work place. It is not to imply that outside of the realm of nursing one cannot do as they wish. There may be stumbling blocks and hurdles to challenge. Nonetheless, proper perseverance and vigilance for changing trends in practice will overcome the pitfalls that the professionally licensed nurse might encounter. As in any of the professions, updating and the honing of one's practice will facilitate professional transitions and communications. This can be accomplished by attending professional continuing education courses and seminars for professional enhancements. Inclusively, participating in community health fairs and online webinars of the nursing specialties and trends. With an ever changing world of new technologies, the professionally licensed nurse will need to keep abreast of what changes may and will occur. Electronic medical record charting and cyber informatics relevant to patient care are some of the newest methods of data collection, patient monitoring and follow up care.

Since the inception of the licensed practical nurse, the role of the licensed nurse has undergone a multitude of changes. Responsibilities have become greater and respectable. Collecting detailed baseline data and patient history will set the primary care information for nursing care. This may include vital signs and an initial family history of health and diseases that may have been experienced by an immediate family member including but not limited to lifestyles of living. Also, traumatic insults that will be conveyed to the professional healthcare teams.

In certain facilities, the professionally licensed nurse may ascertain a physical and psychosocial baseline of data. A full preparation of the patient quarters may be done with the assistance of ancillary personnel. Inclusively, follow up care within the continuum of care from admission to exit of care will be established. Assisting with medical and administrative communications will need to be established with family and significant others on the palate of care. This will be extracted from the patient care record or electronic medical record that will provide the goals for patient instruction of exit nursing care and treatment upon discharge form the facilities. Encouraging the patient/client to adhere to doctor's orders, medication regimens as well as appointments with their doctor and specialty providers. Applications of practical nursing theory have been redesigned to meet the ever-changing role of the licensed practical nurse.

From education to practice and from area of specialization to independent and mobile professionally licensed nursing, a world of healthcare needs can be met. As it was from the beginning, the practical nursing student of today will be tomorrow's frontline healthcare provider. Bridging the gap of the nursing shortage and setting the path to professionally delivered nursing care is the goal and challenge of the professionally licensed nurse. It can be said that the license of the practical nurse is the key to the start a well-rounded approach to healthcare. A turnkey for licensed practical nurses is to be multitalented as well as multidiscipline oriented.

Fearlessly exploring areas that build and strengthen the practice of the licensed practical nurse. Researching areas that expand the role of the licensed practical nurse will broaden the vision of the professionally licensed nurse, from data collection to specialty functions not acquired in the course of classroom preparations. All theories in practical nursing education provide an introduction to the specialties and variations of nursing practice. That is where continuing education and professional enhancement applies to further hone the professionalism of the licensed nurse. From health educator, a data collection specialist or even practicing in the corporate environment. The practice of the professionally licensed nurse is not limited in the areas of pharmaceutical or legal research specialist as well. How far and to what extent the professionally licensed nurse can go will be based on how well founded and prepared the professionally licensed nurse becomes.

In the halls of multidiscipline healthcare are many doors in which professional nursing may enter into. Behind each and every door are multilevel channels of communication, the first level being specialty ready. There are administrative, legal and professional provider team channels that provide professional guidance and direction with professionally licensed nursing practice. As doctors' orders permits the professional licensed practical nurse to collect blood and body fluid specimens. Whereby, collection of these and other specimens provide for analysis, diagnosis and treatment of patient/client conditions. An electrocardiogram may also be obtained, in support of establishing a baseline of primary data that will provide the medical and nursing team with another baseline for patient/client care and treatment. Such data will set the pace and the direction in which each communication turns its focus on delivering efficient and effective professionally licensed nursing care.

Opening the door to the implementation of professionally licensed nursing is not limited to one language but to many who pursue the professional nursing services for mankind, inclusively, specific language being that of culture or of professionals, such as the legal and industrial communities. No one is left out of the process for the delivery of healthcare, bringing a unity on a broader sense. Whether home or abroad, the professional licensed practical nurse has earned his/her name and place in the world of professional healthcare.

There are many professional choices that may open venues through which the licensed nurse may develop professionally. Thereby, accepting the professional challenge, which, may provide a positive venue in which to practice. There, the challenge to step into the doors of professional enhancement and professionalism, whereby, taking on such professional enhancement, new horizons await. All one has to be is dedicated and willing to broaden the horizons that bring readiness to the professionally licensed nurse. Styles of practice may vary, but to shine, stay well polished and tight at the seams. Meaning that, being a mature and well-founded professionally licensed nurse will produce an outstanding, exemplary quality outcome.

It may appear that this is an entry-level area of nursing. In fact it is not. There are certified nurses assistants; home health aides and patient care assistants by which to enter into the professional practice of nursing. Practical nursing, in perspective, is a giant step forward in the direction where ancillary and allied health professionals provide one common goal. That goal is, to provide, with professionalism and dignity, the mind and hands that were educated and trained for those in need of professional nursing and healthcare. We hear, see and empathize to meet those needs efficiently and effectively without prejudice or reservation.

In recognition to the founders of healthcare and nursing, the professional licensed practical nurse, in essence, steps forward and extend their hands, lifting up the integrity of practical nursing, to all in the processes of professional licensed nursing. To children, the parents, and the entire family unit easing the struggles for a happier and healthier tomorrow. Industry and the market places that manufacture and provide the tools with which to deliver such care have also paved the way in which the licensed nurse instrumentally provides. No venue is too big or too small for the dedicated licensed nurse.

On the job education and training in-service and in practice training is an ongoing professional educational process. The licensed nurse may encounter a procedure in which a specific protocol may need to be applied. A team leader, be that a medical doctor or registered nurse, will instruct, with detail, supervise and provide a professional critique at the clinical setting; thereby sharpening the skills and practice of the professionally licensed nurse. Be it a new practice, such as observing and maintaining the functions of an intravenous pump or enteral feeding pump device. Or even specific applications of treatment based care.

Healthcare and practical nursing is a worldwide integration of all of the disciplines of professional healthcare, whether direct and indirect. This unified collaboration of contributors to the healthcare delivery continuum has embraced the profession of practical nursing for over a century. Having been welcomed from all parts of the globe, those who give of their lives for the betterment of the integrated balance of the health and welfare to humanity.

A child awakens to the dream and desire of becoming a helping hand to the ills of the world. While forging his way through life he encounters all the reasons for his pursuits. He looks around and further forms the belief that he can do something. He encounters challenges and jumps the hurdles of peer and community pressure. He develops a plan by which to integrate him self, as part of a team. With guidance and perseverance the child discovers that his dreams and desires can become reality. Of such intenseness, the steps into nursing and healthcare are taken. There may be many influences that hurry the steps. It could be a parent, a family member, a friend or even the family doctor. All in all, while becoming a contributing player in the field of healthcare and professional licensed nursing, the stepping-stones are pursued.

Who would think, that an experience would impact a child or even an adult, at any point in life, how important they are in pursuit of meaningful service to humanity. Such a decision expresses a state of maturity with positive life long affects. To be someone who makes a difference in the lives of others. To become the link in the chain of life that is so needed. To see and experience, that a decision in time has helped so many. This actualization of the dream has brought the rewards from the heavens.

Looking forward to becoming an integral contributor in the work place is an honor in and of itself. Without prejudice or reservation, faithfully delivering quality outstanding professional nursing care. Diligently maturing through the rites de passage of the nursing profession and living the rewards of knowing your patient is treated with a respect beyond words. This professional maturational process builds the foundations that produces a vision of diverse and specialty choices. Where the professionally licensed nurse chooses and serves, with the preparation required, will be welcomed as an accepted member, being the nurse in the work place.

It can be understood that the professionally licensed nurse comes from diverse cultures and traditions. All of which have a common goal. That is, to identify with the pursuit of happiness and the human balance of health and wellbeing. With that in mind, there is an array of psychosocial influences, from cultural, ethnic and religious backgrounds. Although we come from different countries, cultures and traditions, the licensed practical nurse has learned to put all differences aside and tend to humanity and its wellbeing. The professionally licensed nurse, therefore, is able to adapt to various levels of care that leave long lasting impressions on inner city and urban practice. There are areas where the under served will need to be heard and cared for as well. This is where quality of care is performed; by the licensed nurse without prejudice. With compassion and an empathetic approach, as well as an ear for the nursing care recipient, go hand and hand. Applying an objective approach to professionally interpret the subjective inferences of the patient/client being served as well.

The professional approach of practical nursing, healthcare case management and performance depend on the preparation and readiness of the licensed nurse. This is primarily a hands' on documenting practice. The progressive professional nursing skills will need close and detailed attention. Building a well-based professional vocabulary is fundamental, in order to convey the continuum of care. What the professional licensed practical nurse listens to, that is subjectively expressed by the client/patient, and observes, is interpreted objectively in the professional documentation process. Thereby, documenting a subjective expression of what the patient/client experiences into the professional medical-nursing language which is applied to the continuum of professional medical and nursing performance. This professional communication delivers a clear approach to the implementation of healthcare, from a professional standpoint. Therefore, all nurses delivering nursing care to the patient/client will share in this communication. All medical providers will also provide their input and results, which will express in a clear picture that there is continuity of care. Medical doctors further refine how well the professional licensed practical nurse produces professional results, evidenced by the care in and at the clinical work place. By the application of compassion and empathy, the practical nurse will therefore produce a satisfied healthy result throughout the healing process.

These first steps are learned in the classroom with written exercises that build and strengthen a comprehension of the applied professional medical and nursing terminology. But, it is the real exposure and practical application of nursing and medical terminology that sharpens and professionalizes the practical nurses communication, thereby, producing clarity as well as a concreteness to the healthcare continuum. From primary nursing to the intensity of specialty nursing practice, is where the rungs of the continuum are climbed and the heights are reached. The deeper the emersion of practice, the clearer the communications are among the nursing and medical specialties.

From the acquisition of client history, a professional application and treatment can be effectively rendered. The details that apply may vary from client to client. Also, from verbal to non-verbal, as it applies to client/patient treatment and follow up care. Paying close attention to the details upon delivering professional nursing care will result in positive outcomes. Carefully evaluating practical nursing applications with a team approach, the licensed nurse will know how effective and efficient the treatment has been.

No handicap is preventive of the delivery of healthcare. This does not imply unsafe or poor qualitative nursing care. The practical nurse may have a handicap such as an amputation or perhaps a bilateral lower limb amputation. Having a prosthesis or limited use of a limb. Be it a finger or the hand. Nonetheless, this does not impede the learning and nursing care delivery process. Let's say a dismemberment of the foot or hand. Be it a finger or a toe or that of a sense organ occurred. Hopefully not. All of the professional education that the practical nurse has learned can still be applied in practice. The conveyance of collected data can also be professionally delivered. With technology and tool acquisition, there is no limit of information and data impediment. The team approach is what makes the delivery of practical nursing care a professional practice possible.

Progressive professional licensed practical nursing skills performance and communications will need close attention. It is not to imply that the practical nurse is under the microscope, but that reporting accurate results of nursing care will be paramount. Practical nursing is primarily a hands-on nursing practice; the genuine desire and ability for caring with skill for delivering healthcare is all that one needs for a professional team performance. We listen, we learn, and we convey. Case finding and the professional delivery through communicating are contributory in the professional implementation of nursing.

Though the age of the licensed nurse may seem to depict immaturity, such as that of a nineteen year old, it is not a factor; for communicative and complete health care delivery; although, there is an age limit, for the entry-level nurse. Eighteen years of age is the standard requirement for the acquisition of the professional license for practicing as a professionally licensed nurse. There are institutions that a student in high school is able to pursue an education in practical nursing and the allied health careers. The educational halls of those schools have become an integral part of nursing and allied health developments today. Although, licensed practical nurses, from high school, are still in the mainstream of licensed nursing practices; some have gone as far as to become medical doctors, registered nurses, nurse practitioners, health educators, lawyers and then some. To mention a few, further entering the halls of the professions. As diverse as the professions may be, there are many avenues for professional development and practice. Young pro-school graduates, as well as, seasoned pro-school graduates, display an array of the ages, from entry level to well-established practitioners. Professional development through the practice continuum of care is a team goal. Being an integral member of the healthcare delivery team, the licensed practical nurse effectively contributes to the health and well being of the healthcare recipient.

The licensed nurse learns and develops procedures that can be tapered to the needs of the nursing care recipient. This is where the art of practical nursing applies the skills and professionalism that makes the licensed nurse who they are. Protocols are primarily based on the scope of practice, which may be enhanced or limited by institution, community or levels of law. This is not to imply that the licensed practical nurse is totally limited to any practice, as a licensed nurse. It simply states, that depending on various factors of the practicing licensed nurse, the scope of practice may be broad or goal oriented, depending on the professional healthcare delivery team. A school at which a practical nurse practices may be protocol based. The medical doctor will initiate a doctors' order with a standard of care. A registered nurse will review the doctors' orders as per the practices and protocols of the nursing process.

No professionally licensed nurse or student nurse may be autonomous. Except under certain circumstances, where a true licensed nurse decision may have to be made in concurrence with the health care delivery team, the licensed nurse in the workplace will need to follow a standard of care. The standard of care and practice will be expressed by federal, state and local guidelines agencies, which govern scope of practice. (See Nurse Practice Act in your state) and (Board of Regents in your state).

The work place can be an institution such as a hospital, nursing home or rehabilitation facility or even a house of worship. Also a medical office practice but not limited to a trailer, bus or public sites and venues. A trailer may be designed and implemented, as a mobile community medical clinic. Thereby, delivering healthcare to communities where a primary clinic may not exist. Or where a population of people may not be able to get to a medical clinic. This may be a clinic of private practice serving the public of a hospital based outreach medical program. A bus or recreation vehicle may also be converted into a clinic on wheels. Also enabling professional medical and nursing services to be delivered to communities of handicap persons and the under served. Although supervision is needed, be it a licensed medical doctor or a licensed registered nurse, the practical nurse will still need to rely on administrative protocol. The administrative protocol will be in the policy and procedure practice manual of the employing or contracting agency or facility. A nurse's registry or agency will also provide a standard of care and practice description with guidelines and scope of practice. Usually with a licensed medical director and written guidelines.

The registered nurse reviews the doctors' orders, as per the practice and protocols of professional nursing practice. The professional licensed practical nurse also, reviews and implements the doctors' orders, like a gate keeper in practice, applying standards of nursing, via instruments of documentation and communication. A frontline of care by the licensed nurse, as a first responder to patient care, include reviewing all pertinent data relevant to patient/client care. Whether reviewing immunization records, providing immunizations or providing first aid under urgent circumstances.

The licensed practical nurse will communicate with the registered nurse, licensed medical doctor or an emergency medical technician and paramedic, conveying vital information for the continuation of professional medical and nursing care. Whether medical or surgical interventions may be required, the professional licensed practical nurse will be a very necessary and integral member of the healthcare team, as the history of nursing has expressed. The professional licensed practical nurse is not limited to consulting with the registered nurse in an emergency room or obtaining consent to treat, from the patient, parent or guardian ad litem, implied or expressed. When professionally trained, to obtain an electrocardiogram or blood and body fluid specimens, may be procedures that are professionally performed.

The institutional, clinical and community practice, of the professional licensed practical nurse will be implemented through the mission and protocols stated by such clinical policies, laws, rules and regulations. Not withstanding, federal, state, local and community laws relevant to the Nurse Practice Act. The laws and statutes are primarily the same, to review and collect data for the highest quality of care, to establish a baseline in the continuum of nursing care and practices. All professional practitioners have a standard by which to measure and evaluate professional outcomes. Therefore, the professional licensed practical nurse, by implementing such standards of care, provides a pathway that produces a bridge in attaining the common goal.

The cliché, "first impressions are long lasting impressions" applies to all who work in healthcare, therefore, professionalism and preparedness reflects on the work place environment. Yet still another cliché, "a facility is only as good as its staff" may be an indicator that may produce harmony amongst staff, which may be applicable. How well the wheels in motion are oiled can only be depicted by the institutional or clinical performance and outcomes. The welcoming staff expresses professional preparedness. Putting the client first and foremost, illuminates an environment for the delivery of good health and the attainment of a well oiled healthcare delivery nursing team. The introduction of healthcare in a positive and embracing manner, of the client/patient, sends the most professional message; that we the professional licensed practical nurses are integral members of the nursing and medical teams ready to deliver. Therefore, the professional licensed practical nurse projects, radiantly, the warmth of empathy, thereby, understanding the needs of the patient/client. It is paramount that a well groomed, professionally well versed and rounded professional demeanor is expressed.

Many cliché's and statements are born of first impressions, attributes and misattributes as well as misinterpretations. Therefore, a customer, client or patient is not the only recipient of nursing care that may be affected. A family, a community as far as a vast population may define the impressions produced by the quality of care provided.

The recipient of nursing care may also be the employer and the contractor. Be it a facility or an open site where people gather. Wherefore, an employer may be an institution of healthcare, a hospital, a nursing home or a rehabilitation facility. But not limited to healthcare agencies or outsourcing employment healthcare nursing registries or corporate organizations. Whether it is a labor union or a licensed practical nurse association, which represents professional licensed practical nurses, each and every licensed practical nurse represents not only the employer, but also the practices of the professional licensed practical nurse as an integral member of such employer and its member teams.

A trailer, a bus or mobile treatment vehicle may be designated for delivering healthcare services to a community or a specific venue. A hospital or private outreach medical clinic healthcare programs, thereby enabling healthcare services to reach the handicapped the disabled and most importantly, the underserved communities, may deploy this.

The practices of licensed nursing at a venue site, that may be a public event, a concert, the launching of products or services, have a policy relevant to nursing practice. This means that the licensed nurse, under the corporate or professional medical supervision of the event site contractor, will need to be diligent in such practice or service of the event venue responsibilities. To observe, perform and report any and all unusual occurrences are key to a successful event venue practice. The licensed practical nurse will be the first responder at the venue event site or camp. Always being prepared and ready to provide professional nursing care will be paramount. Prevention of untoward occurrences, by observation and communication, will project the readiness of the licensed nurse in the joint effort of a successful event.

On land, sea or air the nurse may need to provide professional nursing care, depending on the circumstances. Under such circumstances, may be to evaluate an occurrence where the mechanism of injury or illness is present to a patient. Be it an accidental trauma or an acquired illness. The situations may vary at a public place, motor vehicle accident site or at the patient's workplace. The licensed nurse may also travel nationally or internationally. Being prepared for this style of professional nursing requires flexibility. Therefore, at this juncture, professional nursing care may present a challenge. Before taking on such a diverse challenge requires being able to adapt and be receptive to change. The professional licensed nurse can acclimate with assistance and follow through respectively. Never be afraid to ask any question or feel intimidated by new surroundings. There will always be a well-rounded team leader to guide the licensed nurse in producing an outstanding outcome. The main focus of practical nursing is promoting the health and well being for all recipients of nursing care. The licensed nurse performs professionally and respectfully to deliver, respectively nursing care, to the recipients. Uniformity and continuity are staple aspects to the communication of the professional nurse. A cohesive team approach is essential to the communication of the professional licensed practical nurse. A cohesive team approach will deliver impeccable and outstanding nursing care and produce healing outcomes to the recipients of professional practical nursing care and their counter parts. From reception to exit of practical nursing care, each and every recipient need be heard and responded to in a professional and meaningful manner.

In the forefront of things, the need for the provision and promoting of healthcare will prove the need for professional licensed practical nursing. Therefore, Homeland Security and the protection of humanity against disease and disaster are also characteristics of what the licensed nurse will contribute in time of peace and tragedy. Casualties of accidents and exposures receive healthcare and guidance to maintain and promote a balance of health. As tumultuous as a happening may be, the professional nurse can adapt and integrate their professional skills to bring comfort to those in need and support within the team approach. In the unselfish performance of the professional nurse and the accomplishments of a professional delivery, the results will yield the outstanding outcomes of the common goal.

In peace time and fragile times, licensed practical/vocational nurses will need to stand firm and always be prepared to deliver outstanding, exemplary, quality nursing care, sometimes at a moments notice. One must try to be well rested and ready to deliver. Burnout prevention is accomplished with good time and stress management. Having an outlet such as exercise, and arts and crafts can divert stressors. Dancing and swimming are terrific outlets. Yoga and stretching are also good exercise. Whichever avenue of release by which to decompress one chooses will contribute to positive morale and readiness.

In a life of great pursuits, one challenges the obstacles of discontent. The battles, as subtle as they seem, bring victory to new moments in each day.

N = Never
U = Underestimate
R = Real
S = Supernatural
E = Empathy

Born of The Soul with Truth
Hard Wired to The Bone

CHAPTER TWO

EDUCATION

J UST WHEN YOU thought school was over, a new chapter
shows up. This chapter brings together all who endeavor in the
art of healing as well as the art of caring. No more pencils. No
more books.... or so you thought. Here, as we practice the art of
caring, new tools and applications will facilitate our practices.

Time is never wasted when things go right.
Not even when things go wrong.

Things done right move forward the learned lessons of the past.
It took a multitude of nurses and medical personnel to move lessons
forward. Each lesson facilitated the weakening of myths, ancient
beliefs, rites and rituals. There are still ancient medical practices
and methods of healing in existence. Life is pretty simple. Life is
only complicated by what is believed and not known. Throughout
life, humanity becomes separated from the simple truth. Therefore,
the licensed nurse is prepared to be up for the challenge, taking on
the rites and rituals head on, that may have affected the weak, the
broken, the ill and infirm. Often and without question, forging on,
in pursuit of comforting the broken, ill and infirm. It would seem
a great and daunting challenge, but a challenge at the heart of all
existence. The challenge being to reduce the stressors that weighs
upon the individual. Thereby, preventing the moving forward with
the intent of lessoning the burden of taking on the intuitive pursuit
of health, happiness and the freedom. Thereby, reducing negative

mind burdening obstacles; allowing for the new challenges while facing existing challenges.

That which appears to be wrong is the challenge of an obstacle, which interfered with what would be right. To challenge the outcomes incurred by an individual, group or culture would result in the pursuit of joy, happiness and health. Only to experience the joy that the patient/client attains with the conquest of what may have resulted in being defeated by illness or brokenness. To see the patient/client eventually return home to be with loved ones.

Professional readiness begins when one makes the decision to provide a service of professional healthcare for a person or persons in need of dynamic professional health care. Be it a physical, emotional or environmental, healthcare readiness, for efficient and effective delivery, will be co-dependent on professional and education preparedness. The primary objective, to provide nursing care or assist with healthcare where a recipient of professional nursing care is limited to the logistical methods and sequential procedures required. The layperson may not know, or fully understand, what the professionally licensed nurses' educational and training process is really all about.

Generally, it is a common thought that "a nurse is a nurse"; that is, that the function of a nurse, especially the professionally educated and licensed nurses, is for the care of the physically infirm. That the nursing care provided by the professionally educated practical nursing student, and licensed nurse is to provide menial task oriented care. That treatments and procedures, as may be ordered by a duly licensed medical doctor should be performed, as ordered. Or, that is delegated by a duly licensed registered nurse, a nurse practitioner, or even by a physician assistant, based on the licensed physician protocol. Also, that the licensed nurse is for the understanding and caring for the ill and infirm. Furthermore, providing rehabilitative and or palliative nursing care on the healthcare continuum biopsychosocially. That is, physical care, along with the balance of mental health including family and social interventions respectively, which may be overlooked. This would mean to understand the principles and practices of licensed practical nursing treatments and applications.

Imagine Grand Central Station on a rush hour or Denver International Airport with an ongoing flight transfer exchange. People scurrying from work through train stations. From train to train, flight to flight. Everyone making headway toward his or her destinations, only to be back the next day and do it again. Everyday having new and different changes on his or her commute including delays and travel adjustments, weather conditions, affecting his or her commute including commuter attitudes. This is only a mild analogy, of what could be chaotic scenarios, of the nursing process.

Inclusively is the prioritization for the endorsement of patient care reports, patient status and progress, diagnosis, medication administrations and treatment outcomes. Patient preparations and the continuance of nursing care is an ongoing process. Professional documentation and communication for and during change of shifts on the nursing continuum. Applied scientific nursing theory in practice, from point of care to point of exit of care, practical nursing theory will be implemented. From doctor's orders to the implementation of the professional nursing process, the licensed nurse evaluates, implements and monitors the principles and practices of the licensed nurse on the nursing continuum. Thereby, providing quality professional nursing problem solving solutions, further maintaining the dignity and comfort of the patient/client.

Usually, this is influenced by the desire to provide nursing and health support, physically and emotionally for a person or group of persons in need of professional nursing services. Without knowing what it would take to provide such quality practical nursing care by the licensed nurse, professional and empathetic professional nursing care would not be accomplished. Inclusive, are the practical nursing students, who are in the process of attaining the professional education and training with the professional guidance and supervision of nursing instructors.

A person or group indigenous to the healthcare delivery system, are not versed in the language of medicine and nursing. They may not comprehend the outcomes, resulting from the performance of nursing care. Those same indigenous persons will need to be cared for by professionally educated, trained and prepared individuals or groups in a practical and sequential way; to understand how and why medical language is applied. The language of medicine and nursing is a privileged and private communication. It protects the rights of the patient/client throughout the healthcare continuum.

The engagement of the vehicle languages will facilitate a comprehensive outcome. The need for professional interpretations will facilitate implementation of nursing care. The common elements of language, that is cultural, traditional, slang and idiomatic, are to be addressed. It can be said; there is a third dimension in which professional licensed practical nurses stands to deliver. The licensed practical nurse may appear to be the unseen and unheard nurse but is an integral professional of the nursing process, nonetheless. This dimension is referred to as the third dimension, the mid third between the licensed medical doctor and the licensed registered nurse. There is no truly unseen outcome of licensed practical nurse practice.

The doctor prescribes an order and both the licensed practical nurse and licensed registered nurse carry out the nursing logistics. Nursing care rendered, therefore, will go through a process and delivered efficiently with effective results. Therefore, for best patient care, all integral members of the healthcare team need to perform and deliver cohesively. "Nursing is the back bone of humanity" the world even the universe." When the professional licensed practical nurse finds his or her place in it. All who receive the practical nursing care rendered will embrace the professional licensed practical nurse.

Teach a recipient of professional nursing service that we care and they will return in response to that care. The professionally licensed nurse presents the knowledge and readiness to provide professional practical nursing services without prejudice or reservation. Application of same language communications, that is, with medical and nursing ease, lay-term to lay response, may encourage the patient/client to be more open should they return. The patient/client, thereby, demonstrating comprehension of professional licensed practical nurse practice.

Teaching and learning is an ongoing process. It is the respiration of readiness. It is the heartbeat of preparedness. The rhythm, in which professional licensed practical nursing performs, is like a well-charged pacemaker that provides a baseline beat on the nursing continuum. Therefore, the licensed practical nurse is concomitant in nursing and healthcare practice, along with all professional practitioners of healthcare.

Schools of practical nursing vary from first impressions of practical nursing to the hard copy institutions of learning. The soft copy is the introduction to the nursing and healthcare commitments, from self-care to caring for others. From a regular healthcare education course or homecare economics courses, the primary courses providing a foresight for performance of care. Therefore, leading to the hardbound venues of professional healthcare and nursing education. Such as, private practical nursing schools, colleges and universities. Thereby, producing the foundations of quality licensed practical nursing. Inasmuch as one prepares on becoming a licensed nurse, will set a well-lit path to the positive and productive practices of the licensed nurse.

The cyber schools are also included for professional healthcare pursuits. In this day and age of digital technology, with computers, laptops, ipads and palm-tech devices, the pathways for practical nursing developments are endless. There may be some economic factors to deal with, but professional developments can be ongoing. There are many and different applications for learning and professionally enhancing the practices of the professional licensed practical nurse.

How we were held and have received immunization inoculations may as well formed how we ourselves were recipients of nursing and healthcare. Not including our first experiences from birth and childhood, which are forgotten experiences, possibly as toddlers. The ongoing learning experiences may remain, as long as we nurture them, by going forward through the maturational process. Everyone has a set of milestones by which we grow and develop. The skills and applications of learning are not the same for everyone. There are individual goals to meet that form the educational accomplishments toward professional developments.

Licensed practical nursing is a compassionate and professionally empathetic health care delivery profession. The educational process, by which the practical nurse is preparing for, is a dual and multifaceted array of professional developments. First and foremost, is the development of the professional vocabulary attained by which to convey the alignment of the healthcare and nursing continuum. The alignment forms the chain of communication between the patient, who is being cared for and an array of healthcare professionals and providers, to meet the healing needs of the patient/client. The professional language is the vehicle by which the patient/client outcomes are measured, throughout the evaluative processes implemented. Therefore, a readiness to deliver practical nursing care, on the primary nursing level, is paramount. Inclusive, in the practical nursing process are the ancillary allied health professionals, such as the certified nurses assistants, phlebotomists and electrocardiograph technicians who are staple to the nursing process.

The art of practical nursing is best described as being able to discern the colors on the canvas of expression. Recognizing the needs of the patient and producing a comprehensible outcome. Therefore, applying oneself compassionately and attaining the ultimate quality of practical nursing care. Be it in the home, the clinical setting, the community and the workplace.

A note on the workplace.
Everywhere, where there is anyone is the workplace.
Be prepared and ready for it.

Preparation for practical/vocational nursing continues by implementing the language of the healthcare professionals. Developing a comprehensive understanding of human anatomy and physiology will strengthen the foundation of professional licensed nursing, thereby, facilitating medical terminology of licensed nursing. Primary practical nursing combined with specialty nursing practice will provide a much clearer view for the professionally licensed nurse.

In these modern and contemporary times, this language will include cyber medical nursing communications. That is, computer based language for learning, evaluating and documenting the implementation and performance of professional licensed practical nursing. There are many computer and application programs of practical nursing. The one that someone chooses should be able to meet the professional standards for delivering proficient nursing care. Although, styles of teaching and learning may vary, from teaching institution to teaching institution, the practicality of the practical nurse profession will be attained. This is measured by the taking and passing of the state board licensing examination for practical nursing. The licensed practical nurse state boards, for the license to practice as a professional licensed practical nurse may vary from state to state, and geographical location of a state including Puerto Rico and the U. S Virgin Islands. That is because the climactic geography and demography vary by country.

A signature thing about practical nursing schools is the curriculum. A well-developed curriculum will produce a well-rounded and licensed nurse, to be able to provide quality professional practical nursing skills. This will initiate rudimentary foundations in practical nursing. Every practical nursing student, taking on the educational challenges for becoming a professionally licensed nurse, may not complete the challenges. But, will eventually find themselves with the knowledge that, at least, they tried. Possibly, with some professional support, they may succeed.

Primary and baseline knowledge is developed with clinical practicum and full days of hands on nursing care and supervision. Side by side, with the licensed professional registered nurse preceptor, instructor, alongside fellow practical nursing students will provide enlightenments to the nursing process. There will be weeks and months of student practical nurse and patient interactions. Thereby, nurturing the development of the world of professional nursing environment and departmental knowledge. Inclusive is the well-rounded practical approach to patient care and classifications of recipients of practical nursing services rendered. With every learning day, full and comprehensive clinical learning experiences, shape the professionally licensed nurse of tomorrow, from medical-surgical nursing, where the patient/client is treated with medication and surgical intervention, through the primary performance of practical nursing and documentation process. Professionally supported with nursing supervision and post nursing conferencing. As a student of practical nursing, each and every learning experience introduces a new awareness, for the road ahead. The rewards are ineffable.

Practical nursing instructors and staff prepare the practical nursing candidate to become a proficient practitioner of professional practical nursing. By applying practical nursing theory with clinical lab practice in the actual care of patients with nursing needs. The specific needs can be met at the bedside, as well as, at the physicians' office, with physical, mental health and emotional support. Whereby, providing preventive nursing care and the promotion of the healing process. Also, assisting with healthcare and counseling, patient teaching, as well as encouraging the patient with independence and self-care. All in all, observing patient care outcomes, documenting in the patient records and team conference reports.

Professional licensed nursing is a multifaceted and multicultural profession. People of many countries and cultures learn to perform nursing services on the primary level. Learning the languages of cultures and customary influences may vary in medical communication, but the nursing and medical language will convey a consistent level of care to the health care recipient. Idiomatic dialect, that is, of English or Spanish and many other languages, also affect the communication aspects of learning and implementing comprehensive practical nursing care and outcomes. By studying and applying the community language, the professionally licensed nurse can build and develop proficiency within the community for the performance of licensed nursing care.

Generally, English combined with international medical language foundations are the basis of nursing and medical language communications. Written, spoken and professionally expressed communications as well as verbal and non-verbal will provide continuity of practice for the licensed practical/vocational nurse. Nursing ease and medical ease communications are also implemented for the recipient of practical nursing care, to facilitate the comprehension of what is being delivered to the healthcare recipient.

The language of medical and nursing ease is communicated objectively and professionally to the non-medically versed recipient person or group. Since the non-medically versed persons or group are persons of subjective communications, that is, they express what they feel, the practical/vocational nurse will need to extract the subjective communication and convert it into the professional objective language of nursing and medical communications. This would be accomplished by collecting vital sign data, such as, the patient temperature, pulse, respirations and blood pressure, inclusive of the chief signs and symptoms. Also acquiring and documenting the patient primary subjective complaint, that is, when a person is experiencing an ailment, the person will express their symptoms as best they can, describing what it is they are feeling, which then, is interpreted by the professional healthcare team objectively. The objective communications are also expressed for other interdisciplinary professionals such as diagnostic, therapeutic and rehabilitative practitioners.

Practical nursing schools may range from high school, private proprietary schools to entry level nursing college career institutions. The entry levels for practical/vocational nursing require a high school diploma or a general education diploma (GED). A foundation language, be it English or Spanish is primary. Since primary language is a vehicle, that is the communication language that will assist in building the fundamentals of practical/vocational nursing practice, process and professional performance, movement between languages will facilitate comprehension of professional licensed practical nursing and medical communications. Practical nursing school entrance examinations will also have to be challenged and passed. Entrance examinations vary from school to school. The primary entrance examination may consist of English comprehension, use of vocabulary and primary sciences.

As with all languages of communications, the written and spoken interpretation of language is paramount for continuity of professional licensed practical nursing care. Therefore, the development of these primers, essential English, math, understanding of biological sciences, that is, primary human anatomy and physiology, sociology, fundamentals of psychology and public speaking produce concrete methods for critical thinking. In order to establish a foundation in practical nursing fundamentals, medical/surgical nursing, pediatric, obstetrics, geriatric and psychiatric practical nursing skills and development, these fundamental elements are staple requisites for the implementation and performance of the professional licensed nursing process.

Professional jargon or terminology, as it is known, is structurally applied to describe or express a condition or situation. The condition, also know as, the description of the physical and mental state of being, may be of a minor acute illness or injury. It could also be the description or interpretation of a chronic illness or condition, depending on the seriousness or gravity of the patient/clients state of health. The condition may need a short-term treatment or a long-term treatment.

Each condition or treatment, whether short term or long term, will require accurate documentation throughout the practical nursing care process. Therefore, maintaining an accurate record of the practical nursing progress and outcomes. Even any situation, be it environmental or behavioral, will need to be professionally and descriptively documented, to assure the balance of healing with positive outcomes. Medical records documentation is a life-long record that will follow the patient throughout his/her life. By having and building a professional knowledge and usage of the professional aspects of nursing and medical documentation, will benefit the patient/client as well as the healthcare delivery team members, thereby, providing professional performance and quality nursing care. Specific anecdotes will be expressed in the chapters that follow these nurses' notes.

Because every patient/client will have unique individual needs, the methods implemented by the licensed nurse will need to be tapered, adjusted and aligned to meet the individual needs of each patient/client. This art of practical nursing will express how and when it is delivered to the recipient of licensed nursing. The platform by which practical nursing care is delivered is a professional one by the well-educated and prepared licensed practical/vocational nurse.

Accredited schools for state licensure and approved health care institutions are congruent. Learning the art of practical nursing varies from academic schools of practical nursing. The locality may also vary from state to state. There are local, county, state and national laws that govern the practice of the licensed nurse. On the west coast and the southern states, the practical nurses title may vary, thereby, to have the title of licensed vocational nurse. Practical nursing courses may also provide specific education and training, which are tapered to the geographical aspects of the demographic environment. Such as, the tropical southern and western regions and or temperate eastern regions in which people live, including Alaska, Puerto Rico and the U. S. Virgin Island of the Caribbean.

The United States Armed Forces, also, have schools for practical/ vocational nursing where national and international practical/ vocational nurses provide a front line of nursing care. The Unified Code of Military Justice governs the military healthcare practical nursing delivery process. These schools are ridged and maintain squared off practical nursing care process high and tight; meaning that the delivery of licensed nursing is from point of need to point of exit procedurally and sequentially has a tightness of professionally accountability. The licensed nurse, in military practice functions with unique military healthcare teams. It can be practicing as a civilian licensed nurse or as a military licensed nurse.

Either way, the Unified Code of Military Justice equally governs the professional performance and responsibilities of the practical/ vocational nurse. Since the Unites States Armed Forces provides healthcare, by and to, all branches of the United States Armed Forces. They are The U.S. Army, The U.S. Navy, The U.S. Marines, The U.S. Air Force and The U.S. Coast Guard. Including and not limited to The Allied military and NATO Forces worldwide. There are prisoners of war from every country that during wartime are also the recipients of quality nursing care. Licensing for the vocational/ practical nurses in the U. S. Military are governed by federal and state boards of regents in conjunction with the Unified Code of Military Justice and The State Department of the United States of America.

Due to the national and international travels of the military licensed practical nurses, many military and local laws will need to be observed. The military licensed nurse will learn about customs and traditions, when practicing abroad, which may be by rank. Depending on whether being stationed on land or at sea, there are also a specific set of rules and regulations that will also need to be observed. As a United States Navy corpsman, I worked and trained alongside military medical personnel, have had to have specific military medical training, in order to provide quality healthcare to military and civilian persons. I have been educated to teach specific nursing and medical care for military personnel and civilians for land, sea, and air and submarine squadrons. That is the most intense type a training the military and civilian nurse could experience. From induction into the United States Navy and Armed Forces, through the enlistment and completion process and exit of military service to the United States of America, an experience of and for a lifetime.

Uniformed schools of nursing may vary from school to school. Signature schools of practical nursing may be private schools or publicly funded government schools. It does not matter, if the school of practical nursing is privately funded or publically funded, the goals are the same. That is, to meet the nursing and healthcare needs of the healthcare recipient therefore the art of practical nursing should be consistent. This continuum prepares the practical nurse in primary and allied areas of healthcare. Each school of practical/vocational nursing, whether it be a college a university, like were the origins of practical nursing education and training, in 1909. Types of uniforms the nursing students wore identified the private or vocational schools. The nursing caps also, had identifying features. Some nurse caps had a design when no stripe was noted. A blue stripe identified the professional licensed practical nurse and other type stripes, such as the plaid stripe identified the specific school of practical nursing from which the practical nurse graduated. Those particular stripes, also, identified the difference between the registered nurse and the practical nurse. Registered nurses wore one or double black stripes. The black stripes were worn to denote a respect and mourning for Florence Nightingale. The shapes and designs of nurses' caps identified the Alma Mata of which nurses graduated from. In these contemporary times, nurses from all nursing schools are not wearing nurse's caps at all. Male nurses never wore nurses' caps. Every level of nursing is not wearing white uniforms. The uniforms have been replaced by either surgical scrub uniforms or colorful uniforms;

like that of pediatric nurses and staff. No uniforms are worn in psychiatric hospitals, wards and clinics. This may be due to the white coat syndrome affect. The white uniforms produce anxiety and possibly emotional disturbances in the psychiatric nursing units. Civilian and regular street clothes, worn by mental health nurses and professionals, may ease the anxiety and fear that psychiatric and emotionally imbalanced persons may experience.

Many mandatory healthcare courses are offered in the continuum. One such course is cardiopulmonary resuscitation, (CPR), a course that will need to be periodically refreshed with annual or biannual training certification. There are also, other continuing educational courses, such as; infection control and prevention also need to be kept up with. As the development of nursing practice unfolds, and greater responsibilities are placed on the nursing profession, more continuing educational responsibilities will need to be maintained. Such as, child abuse, elder abuse, domestic violence and the legal aspects of nursing practices. With the basic and technical steps always in motion, continually attending professional workshops and seminars for professional licensed practical nursing updates. No one needs to carry around unwanted bacteria and hitch hiking viruses to interrupt the healthcare continuum and the delivery of outstanding healthcare by professional licensed nursing.

Continuing education is a good path to follow, in that changes and accountability of those changes need to be kept abreast of, periodically and frequently. Professional seminars, relative to the allied health professions are also offered for the licensed nurse. By doing so, keeping up to date is absolutely necessary for the advancement and practice of quality professional nursing. The licensed nurse performs healthcare teaching as well, from point of care to point of exit. With climbing the professional ladder and having a well-rounded knowledge of the nursing profession, the licensed nurse can also become a teacher or an adjunct instructor of the allied health professions. There is a growing need for competent instructors of allied and ancillary healthcare providers. This means that the spectrum of care has broadened the role of the professional licensed nurse. Whether for private proprietary schools of allied health or higher institutions of learning, such as, colleges and universities, the need can be met. Thereby, becoming a strong rung on the ladder of the healthcare delivery continuum, forthwith. For God and Country I will serve my fellow man willingly.

CHAPTER THREE

CHOOSING AN AREA OF PRACTICE

I T IS AMAZING, when the practical nurse, after successfully graduating from the school or the university of practical nursing, will have so many options from which to practice at. The world and everyone in it have embraced students of practical nursing, who by choosing to endeavor and further their careers' will become outstanding professionally licensed nurses. Upon the successful completion and attainment of the license to practice as a licensed nurse, blessings await in this rewarding practical nursing profession. When a patient/client is provided with such professional clinical, bedside and the personal attention to detail that each patient/client receives, the rewards are beyond words. Upon entering into the many levels of specialty clinical settings, it is an amazing experience of how and when the patient/client have welcomed the practical nurse.

It actually takes a well-founded baseline of professional maturity and professional comportment that produces such positive healing and outcomes; when the licensed nurse performs. With the leap of faith and the welcoming support of all healthcare and nursing team members, there could only be such a harmonious outcome. No one is perfect, but with professional efforts for producing such outstanding and positive outcomes, the licensed nurse will perform in an exemplary manner. Therefore, becoming recognized as an exemplary professional, delivering outstanding healthcare, without reservation, the professional care of each and every client/patient is a staple signature of the licensed practical nurse. The licensed practical nurse has made his/her mark, throughout the practice of nursing, in every clinical setting worldwide. The areas in which the licensed nurse may also apply theories in professional healthcare can be expressed in the teaching of perspective nursing and healthcare candidates as well.

After experiencing more than forty years of teaching, throughout the allied health fields, has kept me up to date in the practices of healthcare. The many varieties of healthcare including providers of healthcare equipment, the possibilities are endless, where the professional licensed practical nurse may choose to practice at. By endeavoring to integrate into a particular area of professional healthcare, thereby, taking the initiative to perform at a clinical setting would make for having the confidence to perform efficiently and effectively.

The implementing of computers together with technology, along with every healthcare entity has facilitated the caring and healing outcomes of the patient/client. Social media and communication applications have also played a major role in how a patient/client receives professional licensed nursing care. Pharmaceutical companies and providers of durable medical equipment (DME) have become significant partners with the medical, surgical and nursing professions, each one having a significant role in the delivery of professional healthcare services. Pharmaceutical companies or pharmacies provide therapeutic medications as ordered by the licensed medical doctor, and surgical supply companies provide pre or post-surgical equipment and devices for therapeutics implementation. Also, the DME suppliers providing therapeutic equipment and devices, such as, hospital beds, walkers or wheel chairs, but not limited to diabetic products and expendable products. The vehicles applied in the concerted efforts to meet patient/client needs have bridged gaps throughout the healthcare delivery system.

The journey of the professionally licensed nurse toward integrating into the nursing profession will fare through many multifaceted aspects of healthcare. There are licensed practical/

vocational nurses that may choose to practice only in the general areas of nursing. That seems a favored comfort zone. Don't get too comfortable because things will change, there too. There are, also, professional nurses that are eager to explore other medical and nursing areas of healthcare. This can be from pediatrics to geriatrics and all other areas in between. The in between areas will involve stepping up and into required preparation for the chosen medical and nursing specialty. Preparations for the chosen specialization of practice may also require immersion of studies such as variations of research in order to professionally comprehend the logistics of such practice. Logistically, this is, to know the applications of specialty communication components and successful follow through. To know and understand the how and why of the nursing applications of the practices of professional licensed practical nurse, exists the outcomes throughout the healthcare continuum.

Specializations in nursing have evolved into a global spectrum, due to the shortage of registered nurses and licensed practical nurse providers, within the healthcare delivery system. Professional attrition and the many changes to the medical and nursing professions have taken its toll, not only on the professional practices of nursing, but on every healthcare community worldwide. There is an immense nursing and allied healthcare gap. To bridge or close that gap and the shortage of quality professional licensed nursing, becoming an integral member amongst the broad horizon of healthcare providers is a choice to be made. No matter what any other constituency, of the healthcare workforce, may say or attempt, there will always be the need for professional licensed nurses. The professional practical nurse is here to stay. Always keeping up with the changing times, and assisting with the long and the short of the healthcare gap and vast nursing shortage. That void will be met with fervent professionalism. Taking on greater and meaningful responsibilities. To think that cyber nurses note communication at a health facility and in the fields of healthcare was not far fetched. All nurses need to flow with the times. Though the logistical economics may not always be there, the licensed practical nurse can integrate for the balance.

The times have changed. People are living longer. Healthcare has become expensive. The inclusion of the professional licensed practical nurse amongst every area of the specialties in medicine and nursing will provide for the balance of affordable healthcare. The economical factors will bring bedside, clinical, community and even school nursing right to the patient in any variation of licensed nursing. Therefore, taking on new and broader responsibilities will have the professionally licensed nurse ever moving forward on the healthcare continuum.

The entry level into the medical/surgical specialties of nursing practice is primarily based on clinical experience and development thereof. Combined with professional enhancements courses, such as, the addition of the twelve lead electrocardiograph technician for acquiring a twelve lead electrocardiogram, which assists with diagnosis and treatment of patients with cardiac conditions. Clinical implementation of telemetry monitoring of the patient/client with cardiovascular diseases can optimize professional medical and nursing outcomes. Obtaining the professional certification as a phlebotomist makes the professional licensed practical nurse an asset. Thereby, assisting in acquiring laboratory blood specimens for diagnostic procedures and the treatment of specific illnesses and diseases. There are so many levels of professional enhancements by which the licensed nurse may choose from up to advanced practices. Preparation and study for the professional enhancements and becoming certified in those professional enhancements, which apply to your chosen specialty, where professional nursing may be practiced, is an endeavor in and of itself.

The licensed nurse will, eventually, develop a broader and practicing knowledge of the spectrum of specialties. Whereby, implementing professional theory in practice, along with attending and participating in healthcare specialty seminars and workshops, will help to further advance specific specialty practices in licensed practical nursing. The umbrella by which the undertaking of professional development and practice occurs will depend on the policies and procedures granted to the scope of practice within the legal guidelines of the licensed nurse. The flexibility of those guidelines will also rest on the professionally licensed medical community. The compliance factors may also be implemented through legislation throughout the nation, states and communities where the specialty practice of the licensed nurse, which may be required.

Where and how does the licensed practical nurse fit may seem like almost an unanswerable feat for some providers of logistical healthcare providers. The answer is clear. All areas of healthcare will need the professional licensed practical nurse to ease immediate and frontline services for consumers of healthcare. Frontline practical nursing, such as under the direct supervision of a licensed medical doctor, in a community setting or event may be the start of such independent practices of the professional licensed practical nurse. There may be open, public and or private clinical, settings where health data collection may occur. This may be where by performing procedures like measuring and or monitoring of vital signs. Also, acquiring specific specimens from patient/client body fluids for specific diagnostic procedures. Diagnostic procedures may be acquired for any specific specialty, the likes of, geriatrics; pediatrics, maternal and child care as well as oncology, to name a few. There are cardiovascular, orthopedic, dermatology and an array of surgical specialties and professional medical practices, where the professional licensed practical nurse may perform professional medical and surgical assistance. The versatility of professional licensed nursing can be endless, when contributing to the health and welfare of humanity.

The educational preparation and training provide all rules of thumb for professional licensing and acclimation into the healthcare delivery system. Therefore, where practice is introduced will present the essential tools of the profession along with the orientation of application and practice for which those tools are expressed. The meet and greet of recipients of professional nursing care and services are the first step components. At that time, an introduction to the necessary tools, such as, writing instruments like the paper and pen, also the electronic components, especially forms and formats. The recording on to medical records in conjunction with the assistance of computers and flow sheet instruments will be the most useful of tracking and monitoring tools. Also, ongoing professional development of staff continually updating in the professional practice of licensed nursing will insure a continuity of professional communications, moving forward.

Bridging healthcare and nursing care between clients and the professions is where the need for professional licensed nursing will always advance. With the necessary assistance of ancillary personnel, such as, certified nurses assistants (CNA), patient care technician (PCT), phlebotomist (CPT) and electrocardiographic technicians (CET), are also integral members of the medical and surgical specialty practitioners. Where one hand reaches for assistance, the licensed nurse extends their hands to keep bridges open and secure for continuity of the practice of professional healthcare services. All recipients of healthcare will need a gatekeeper that demonstrates care and professionalism. Compassion and empathy are some of most important signature components of the licensed nurse. These component practices are truly demonstrative of the quality of care provided by the professional licensed practical nurse. They make up the cohesive links in the chain of professional nursing care; like the rungs of the human genome, cohesive and sequential, through each and every stage of professional development. Thereby, producing great and positive outcomes throughout the healthcare continuum. A multitude of patients will also be demonstrative of such positive and outstanding outcomes. No on is perfect, but the exemplary performance of the professionally licensed nurse will endure its challenges in every specialty taken on by the professional nurse.

The great demand for quality professional nurses is continually being procured for the medical and surgical specialties. This procurement may be for a clinic, a community or at any level of healthcare institutions.

With the human race living longer and an understanding of old and new illness and diseases, licensed practical/vocational nursing has also entered into independent practice as well. With the advent of higher education, lending itself to the guiding and service of professional licensed nursing, an insurmountable array of challenges can be accomplished. Although a licensed medical doctor or a licensed registered nurse will be required for supervision of the licensed practical nursing team, no professional healthcare challenge can be too small or too great. Being confident in knowing what to do, as a specialty-licensed nurse is essential. Refining the licensed nursing practice means being thoroughly prepared to take on new and challenging professional responsibilities. Research is the foundation of continued preparedness in the professional medical surgical nursing specialties. This begins after completion of required practical nursing curricula, nursing licensure and acceptance or employment for specialty licensed nursing, but may commence sooner.

Every area of health care can be considered a specialty, from medical offices to institutional practice, including corporate, industrial and military nursing. Let's take into account pace practice in nursing. Pace practice is based on particular patient/client scheduling and timed visits. This type of paced practice can be unpredictable at times. So moving right along, the flow of patient/clients and the type and methods of treatments and procedures may dictate the allotment of time per patient/client, per treatment and procedures rendered. This is where every nurse, as an integral team member, performs hands on nursing care to the nursing recipients and follows through by evaluating the steps processed qualitatively. Quantitative nursing care is usually divided by the size of the nursing team. Therefore, a good and strong foundation that you choose is paramount to the outcomes for the recipient of professional nursing care. Administratively, the availability of equipment and essentials will also affect the quality of nursing care performed for the professional nursing recipient.

Areas of interest may not be for every professionally licensed nurse, with medical offices being the broadest of all professional medical practices. Some areas are exciting and action packed with non-stop recipient care profile treatments and procedures. Diagnosis verses preparation to delivery may present a challenge to a specialty of health care practice. Whether medical or surgical, there are also psychiatric applications to a specialty. Providing comfort with an empathetic approach can ease the challenge, but theoretically, it is the sequential procedure, which compliments the professional performance of nursing care to the healthcare recipient. Beginning with the licensed medical doctor, along with other licensed medical practitioners, to the medical office assistant. There are also, certified clinical medical assistants that are required to cross over from one area of the medical office or clinic, as well as, surgical office or clinic, where versatility and flexibility is paramount.

Always keep in mind that the work place is primarily designed, first and foremost, for the medical and or surgical care of the patient/ client and the professional practice by each member of the health care delivery team. There are electronic monitors, computerized telemetry, pulseoxymeter devices and electric vital sign measuring and monitoring devices. Certain areas of professional medical and nursing practice may also be separated by the need of care performed by the licensed nurse for the healthcare recipient. Beginning with frontline nursing intake, performing triage, that is, the acquisition of the patient medical and surgical history and assessment of customer nursing service needs. Not to confuse frontline nursing with front end nursing practice, the area at a particular healthcare setting may be where the patient is received. That would be the reception area where primary healthcare data is acquired, such as, their personal history and demographics or medical coverage. The frontline may be an area of a clinical setting where the patient may be experiencing an acute or chronic illness. Also, where a patient may have experienced a trauma needing immediate medical and nursing attention.

The clinical setting at which the professional nurse practices, will mean that a certain degree of professional flexibility and knowledge will be essential. This is where meticulous and accurate data acquisition and evaluation are paramount towards the efficient and effective diagnosis and treatment of the client/patient. This professional evaluation process, from the onset of professional nursing care, to the exit of professional nursing care, need to be addressed with close attention to details. By doing so, may also include patient teaching and counseling with patient/client participation.

Gathering data for case management and professional applications will mean knowing how to collect and present such data and to which professional organization the data is being collected for. Maintaining and protecting the privacy of the recipient of professional licensed practical nursing care is of utmost importance. This ensures the accurate efficient and effective continuity of providing meaningful professional nursing care and services for clients of healthcare. Thereby, providing return requests from the recipients of healthcare in their continued endeavor for an optimal balance of health. The scales by which the balances are measured are dependent on the maintenance of these measures. Professional developments within the licensed nursing areas, continuing education, communications updating and the array of measures, keep professional pursuits aligned with the continuity of providing exemplary professional nursing services.

Although the clock does not move as fast as the patient/client care process, it is essential that the required tools and instruments be utilized efficiently. Time management in the specialty areas of practice is a key factor in the effective delivery of the healthcare process. All in all, with the expertise of the well-founded professional nurse, healthcare teams can flow effectively.

From when the classroom delivers to when the professional nurse is born is only the beginning of when the choice to practice at a particular place and area is given light. I have started from beginning and from when the choice to practice at a particular medical and specialty clinical areas have helped me to achieved the vision for the specialty practices that I have chosen. I have been motivated from being exposed to professional medical environments. There, I envisioned myself a team member caring for persons and interfacing with professionals of the medical/surgical nursing team. Some specialty areas have been exciting, such as, the emergency rooms, operation rooms, labor and delivery areas or even pediatric units. There were military medical and surgical specialties. There were combat land, air and sea areas, which have medical and surgical specialties within. With the vast areas of practices, a need to bridge and provide healthcare can always begin at the level of professional licensed practical nursing. The expertise developed for the areas that one may choose will need nurturing. Teaching and learning go hand in hand with theses developments.

There are many levels of medical/surgical specialties. Each of these levels has their own medical languages and specialty codes, which sets them apart from similar specialty practice. Since the human body is comprised of a complex of atoms, molecules, chemicals, genes, cells, tissues organs and systems, so are the medical and surgical specialties that provide a complex system of professional healthcare providers. No two or more people will ever have an exact same state of health as another human being. No two or more human beings will have the exact or same illness or disease as another human being. Because the human genome is unique. Therefore, data acquisition for accurate medical and surgical specialty diagnostics and treatments will always vary from one human being to another, definitively, maintaining that all human beings are different.

Wherefore, also, the policies, procedures and protocol may not be the same. There may be similarities, but, nonetheless may be tailored for each and every client/patient. This is where the licensed nurse will need to become familiar with and apply the policies, procedures and protocols in professional practices per client/patient. Eventually, producing positive outcomes throughout the patient/client healthcare and nursing process. Inasmuch as the specialty jargon of professional medical terminology and the medical codes which, may apply.

Every area of medical or surgical specialty will have policies, procedures and protocols which are regulated and governed by National, Federal, State and local laws. There are international laws, rules and regulations as well as international policies, procedures and protocols that may also apply, such as those of the Centers for Disease Control (CDC) and the World Health Organization (WHO). Certain legal statutes may apply as well as the Uniform Commercial Codes of practice. These laws, rules and regulations are designed in the best interest for quality and continuity of the healthcare recipients.

In the corporate practice of licensed nursing, are rigid policies, procedures and protocols. (See the corporate chain of command and communications of the your corporate choice of professional licensed practical nurse practices). All nurses, in general, are continuously updating their theory of nursing practice. There are nursing laws that are mandated for all licensed nurses. Mandates may differ from state to state and from level of nursing practice to level of nursing practice. As a rule, the licensed professional nurse must, by law, maintain professional nursing updates, in order to continue in the practice of professional nursing. It is mandatory.

Note: What may be practiced at one area of a professional medical or surgical specialty area of practice may not apply to another area or institution of the same or similar specialty. (See, also, legal aspects of professional licensed practical nursing in your state).

CHAPTER FOUR

PROFESSIONAL ENHANCEMENTS

Are You Ready?

READY OR NOT may not always apply to professional development. To be certified or not to be certified, also, may not apply. What it takes to be professionally certified for nursing practice at a specialty medical or surgical clinical setting may be a matter of what may be required to practice at such specialty. In a general clinical setting, such as, a family practice medical office or clinic, obtaining certifications in phlebotomy and electrocardiography may suffice. Some professional licensed practical nurses are educationally ready for practice in the specialties of nursing and some are not. The professionally licensed nurse that is ready to practice at a particular medical or surgical specialty may have already taken allied health courses in lieu of having anticipated moving forward in the realm of professional nursing developments. Nonetheless, orientation and exposure to the chosen specialty is paramount. Ask yourself "what specialty should I pick?" and what will it take to practice at that work place? Being clear and diligent is what it would take to make this decision. Just because and area of medical and healthcare practice may appear appealing does not mean that one should make such an unprepared decision. Some nurses see a chosen clinical setting as a "calling", and some nurses prepare for a specific clinical setting as a matter of professional maturation. Which may be expressed as broadening the performance and professional practice of the professional licensed practical nurse. Whatever the interpretation of how the choice is made, one should be prepared for what may be required at the clinical setting in which to practice professional licensed practical nursing.

Do a diligent research on the chosen area that the practice of professional nursing may be applied at. For example, the medical practice at the office of the cardiologist, do require that the licensed practical nurse be professionally trained and nationally certified in performing electrocardiography (EKG/ECG). Thereby, having an understanding of how to recognize the difference between the normal electrocardiogram (EKG/ECG) and an abnormal electrocardiogram. It is of the utmost importance for the licensed practical nurse to be able to recognize the difference between the normal or baseline cardiac rhythm of the patient. Therefore, by recognizing the difference between an arrhythmia, or an abnormal cardiac rhythm, and a dysrhythmia, that is, when a patients' heart is having a difficult or stressful and painful cardiac event. It would be of great and paramount importance of how and when, as well as, who to notify, when such an episode occurs. To acquire an electrocardiogram from a patient would be a non-invasive procedure. No poking no pain.

The same applies, when being professionally trained in any of the allied health adjunct specialties. Becoming a phlebotomist, specifically trained and prepared in acquiring blood specimens is an invasive procedure. Which is the professional act of inserting a special needle into a patients' vein to obtain blood samples. In the practice of phlebotomy, it is, also, important to know when and how to obtain the collection of blood samples, such as, the theory of devices for the drawing of blood samples from the patient and knowing the order of the draw. This specialty education and training will include a thorough understanding of blood sample tube colors and at what laboratory the blood samples are tested and examined. Special education and training of the insertion of an intravenous needle for therapeutic treatments is an invasive procedure. Becoming familiar with the type of blood sample required for any specific medical/surgical clinical setting that the professional licensed practical nurse may chose to practice at will help in how to prepare for such practice.

Explore the professional growth and developments of the nursing and medical communities. Join professional healthcare organizations where you may find yourself practicing at. If you are keeping up with how the proliferation of nursing practices are developing, it could make your decision all the more concrete. There are over two hundred plus medical and surgical specialty areas of practice to date. From information technology nursing to actual hands on bedside and clinical professional licensed practical nursing. Nursing and medical informatics are specialties in and of themselves, from nursing and medical research to reviewing of medical records. For example, reviewing medical records for the clinical management of a patients' health.

These reviews may also include clinical risk groups (CRG), such as, diagnostics, which apply to patient with diabetes mellitus, patients with cardiovascular, cardiopulmonary risk illness and patients with various chronic illness and diseases. There are health evaluation data implementation set reviews (HEDIS) that are monitored by the nursing counsel of quality service (NCQS), Medicaid and Medicare Services (MSS) that are monitored by the Social Security Administration. With a specific type and level of training, the professional licensed practical nurse can acclimate into these specialty areas. Specialized training in computerized medical and nursing informatics may also change periodically and frequently. Therefore, for every season of medical records review, education and training updates are implemented. These types of medical record reviews go through a very lengthy and detailed process. After all, a complete and total medical review of the patient's medical care will help in the healthcare and health management of the patient.

Not everyone is cut out or appropriately prepared for making such a decision, when wanting to change from area of nursing practice to area of nursing practice. While studying to become a professional licensed practical nurse, the practical nursing student will be introduced to the many facets of medicine and nursing. Through the learning and developmental process, the practical nursing student may become attracted to any of the medical/surgical nursing areas for which to practice at. Therefore, be as diligent as you can, in the pursuit of landing your best area for professional licensed practical nursing.

You already graduated from an accredited school of practical nursing. You have successfully passed the state board of licensed practical nursing examination. Of all you have learned at the school of practical nursing, only one question needs to be answered. Am I ready for a specialty? Or should I stay at one place until I retire? Decisions, decisions, decisions. How does the practicing professional licensed practical nurse decide as to what clinical area of professional licensed practical nursing to practice at and for? That decision will depend on if the professional licensed practical nurse is where they need to be or if there is a need to move on.

Health care is an ever changing and challenging profession. Professional licensed practical nursing is on the frontline to these changes. Throughout the professional practice of the licensed practical nurse, there will be changes and challenges. Some changes may be as a result of delegation of patient-care. The requisites of in depth theory of nursing practices may result in the elimination of particular licensed practical nursing responsibilities and/or the addition of licensed practical nursing responsibilities. There are certain nursing assignments that may be delegated to other allied health team members. Such responsibilities may be delegated to the certified nurses assistant (CNA) or the patient care technician (PCT). This makes being prepared an on going process.

By the implementation of technology, technological hardware and software will include becoming familiar or being specially educated and trained in the jargon language complementary and principal to working with the cyber nursing process. We have all heard the Cliché' "easier said than done", well not really. Bearing in mind that a delivery system cannot move any faster than the wheels can turn it. Therefore, being over prepared may be the same as being under prepared. Practical nursing mistakes can occur at any level of licensed practical nursing. So as not to suffer from information overload, keep in mind the scope of practice for the professional licensed practical nurse. This will always have you knowing what to do, rather than falling to being told what to do, where mistakes may occur. Understanding professional boundaries and limitations of the professional licensed practical nurse will assist with keeping within the scope of practice, as a professional licensed practical nurse.

Professional enhancements may prepare the professionally licensed nurse in the work place to better understand the functions of each member of the healthcare team. With the proliferation of nursing informatics, it is essential that all nurses become educated in the implementation of the computer and digital tools that apply within the professional healthcare setting. These tools can be a digital glucometer, a digital tablet for receiving and transmitting patient orders, patient treatments and procedures and the monitoring of medications administration. Electronic medical records (EMR) are maintained, with the inclusion of many interdisciplinary departments, such as medical laboratory orders and results, X-ray and medical imaging reports, social services and many other medical and nursing inter-departmental records. Paper documentation is still essential and complimented by digital application and monitoring of the documentation and implementation process. Write your primary nursing notes on paper and be very sure those notes apply appropriately to each patient the practical nursing care is performed for. Evaluate your practical nursing care as you are implementing the steps that apply throughout the nursing process. Thereby, the quality of care will express positive outcomes that professional educational enhancement are intended to produce.

Professional nursing educational enhancements provides the primary and terminal objectives that produce these positive outcomes. From patient teaching to public speaking, whatever it takes to stay sharp throughout the practice of professional licensed practical nursing will be an ongoing process. Keeping up-to-date with nursing and medical practices, especially when some healthcare practices and application become outdated or enhanced, will be paramount. Furthering the practices of the practical nursing profession, throughout the spectrum of practical nursing, is ever-changing the way people are cared for.

A team is only as prepared as the least prepared member only applies, when communication is as clear and as concrete the communication can be. Each member of the healthcare team are required to be certified and or licensed in the roles that they are responsible for. One such certification, for all practitioners of healthcare, in every area of healthcare, without exception, at professional, private or public settings is being always updated and prepared about the professional trends and application of cardiopulmonary resuscitation (CPR). This is the basic life support (BLS) training course mandated by the Department of Professional Licensing. (See the CPR/BLS requisites of your state). Advanced cardiopulmonary life support (ACLS) training courses may also be required, depending on the professional advancement practices of the healthcare teams, where the professional licensed practical nurse is advancing at. In the advent of advancing in the areas of critical care, such as, the emergency and trauma departments, other professional enhancements may also be required.

Professional enhancements may be offered and attained at the workplace, where the necessity for the advanced professional licensed practicing nursing performance is required. After being introduced to the generalities and general clinical settings, there will be the need for professional development of licensed practical nursing. The primary lessons learned while acclimating into the practice of professional licensed nursing are just a mere glimpse of what happens at particular clinical healthcare settings. There are front end and frontline preparations. Whereas, at some medical clinical and public setting have certain logistical processes that produce a balanced flow of patient care. These logistics, such as, when a patient/client arrive at a clinical setting, will determine if the patient/client is or will be treated for an acute or chronic illness or disease. This will most likely be front-end care, usually at a medical office or clinic, where the registration of preliminary information is acquired. Thereby, verifying the level of eligibility for healthcare and the continuity of healthcare to be provided. The mid-end of licensed practical nursing will occur during the triage and treatment phase of patient care. Follow through logistics may continue from point of care with the application of particular procedures and the acquisition of results from particular diagnostic procedures, such as the use of a glucometer for testing a patients blood glucose levels.

No nursing school or program, teaches advanced practices in nursing. Through the process of continuing professional healthcare education is how the enhancements of career practice are attained. When the certification of an enhancement is achieved, keeping abreast of new developments for continuance of practice will be necessary, in order to provide quality and outstanding patient/client care. During and throughout the learning process, on becoming a professional licensed practical nurse, there are diagnostic procedures that are taught by specialty and allied health programs. With the advent of the Internet, changes in theory and application of newer treatments and procedures, the professional licensed practical nurse can be kept updated. As a matter of ordering such specialized diagnostic tests by the licensed medical doctor, the in depth theory for the practicing of any detailed diagnostic procedure, such as, drawing of blood or obtaining an electrocardiogram, are attained at a school of continuing education for allied health. A certain amount of hours of theory and practice are required for the completion and certification of such allied health programs. A certain amount of contact hours are allotted to theory of the specialty equipment and medical terminology that may be applied to a particular acquisition of specimen and results from a diagnostic procedure for the general or healthcare specialty. Many books, literature and computer apps are frequently published on the allied health education and training programs, also.

Professional organizations of healthcare providers may also provide updated information that would assist with additional required updates. Manufacturer's of medical products and devices may also be contacted for any literature on medical or surgical as well as durable medical equipment that may be used in the healthcare field, particularly, medical products or medical equipment that affect the practice and delivery of quality patient care. Many manufactures of healthcare products, medical equipment, medical devices and pharmaceutical have ongoing seminars about their products as well. Attending professional medical seminars may be one of the best means to staying abreast of changes in reference to the applications of such products. This is because there are professional interactions with the representative of the organizations and manufacturer's of such products and services.

After being trained in the theory, usage and practice of the application of certain allied health courses, a certification examination will need to be challenged. There may be three parts to this process. After passing the theoretical and practical components, additional recertification examinations will be required. These recertification examinations are administered biannually. (See the recertification policies in your state). The primary objectives for recertification are because changes of theory and practice are updated and occur throughout the practices of any and all allied health professional practices. As with much theory and practice of any or all professions, some theory may become outdated and new theory may become amended to be inclusive. As human life styles evolve, products and performance of products may change or may be integrated for maximal and optimal performance, thereby, producing quality medical/surgical therapeutic and nursing outcomes. Through the development of professionally licensed nursing and the professional enhancements of the practices of the licensed practical nurse, a better quality performance of licensed practical nursing care is ascertained.

There are various private, public, colleges, organizations and university schools offering advanced courses of allied health certification. That is primarily where an in depth knowledge of such professional enhancements provide classroom theory and clinical laboratory practice. Each course may introduce the various equipment and devices that may be used in the performance of delivering quality practice of patient care. Because of the varied styles and methods by educators and educational institutions, the applications of theory and practice may be specifically tailored. There are basic, primary and to some degree, in depth clear theoretical applications of how to accomplish the professional performance of quality care. Advancements and new discoveries in healthcare are always happening. Professional healthcare theorists may discover newer and more optimal methods for applying theory of a method or medical devices that may produce optimal outcomes in healthcare. The professional licensed practical nurse may also discover, through application of such theories and professional practices, that not all recipients of nursing and healthcare respond equally to the applications of medical products and medical devices. Thereby, contributing a vast of knowledge about such medical products, medical equipment and therapeutic devices. As is customary, documentation, documentation, documentation on the applications of such medical products, medical equipment and medical devices is paramount for the performance of quality patient/client care. To obtain the most optimal results and outcomes, diligence to the practice of professional licensed practical nursing is paramount.

Never try to carry the whole world on your shoulders. Everyone is a world and everyone is a universe. The constellation of planets and stars within the cosmos denotes that because of such individuality, humanity and all that encompasses the human race is unique. Therefore, the professional licensed practical nursing care provided for every individual will be unique. The results and outcomes will also be unique. So then, the professional licensed practical nurse will provide such unique care to each and every recipient of practical/vocational nursing. This unique care will be accomplished, because as an integral member of the healthcare delivery team, with the appropriate levels of education and training, quality professional licensed practical nursing outcomes can be achieved, for the outstanding performance of healthcare to the patient/client for which the attainment of optimal quality of life can also be achieved.

Factors to be aware of are time and stress management. The best and optimal methods are unique to every professional licensed practical nurse. When practiced, the calm of empathy may be experienced and expressed. Every recipient of healthcare may have the expectation that nurses have a calming and assuring affect just waiting for them. That it is the responsibility of the nurse to get the patient/client to feel that everything will be OK. Well, only a cohesive, well-educated and trained staff can accomplish that. Mostly, every patient/client will experience a level of anxiety or emotional imbalance when faced with an illness, trauma or disease. It could be from the common cold, a trauma, disease or an emotional experience. When the professional licensed practical nurse is prepared, the management of such time will reduce the pressure of stress. That is, professional and personal stress produced in any situation. After all, professional licensed practical nurses are human. There are no bionic humans, in reality. For this reason all areas of nursing for the practice of professional licensed practical nursing should be addressed, from pre-practice to actual and post practice.

In order to self evaluate, the professional licensed practical nurse should keep abreast with current trends and changing protocols. Professional trends and protocols have time factors within them. Therefore, how and when the applications of specific trends and specific protocols should be evaluated, for the appropriate allotments of time per patient/client. Not every patient/client may respond equally to the applications of such trends and protocols. This may affect how time is managed for the quality outcomes of patient/client care. At the end of the day, positive quality affects and outcomes are the goals. In that pursuit, the professional licensed practical nurse would like to get home feeling the sense of accomplishment in their practice as a professionally licensed nurse.

It may not be too far in time before we see interplanetary nursing trends. But nuclear nursing and space travel nursing are not far behind. Keeping our feet well planted on the earthly professional nursing goals is a matter of a forward passage. We may think, not in our lifetime, but it is truly futuristic. As this book is being published, the formation of The United States of America Space Force is becoming a reality. There will be a plethora of additions and changes of the practice of professional licensed practical nursing. There are available openings and offerings for the professional licensed practical nurse that may have great and positive outcomes from their contributions to the unknowns of space nursing practice. A Real First of its kind. New possibilities. Are you ready? Ready or not, the new possibilities of space trends, practices and protocols have arrived. And the professional licensed practical nurse will be prepared for such undertaking. It may seem ridiculous but ever since man has walked on the moon, the preparations that took place before send a human being into space involved specific health monitoring.

No one would ever have imagined that astronauts in space would have their vital signs and health status monitored from earth. With the advent of space stations, the health status of anyone in space would be monitored from this planet earth. Presently, as these notes are being read, people are preparing for trips into space. Satellites have been launched into outer space for decades. Now, there seems to be a growing confidence that human beings would like to take short space trips. As this book is being read, the U. S Navy is conducting Space school training.

There could only be, at this time, the knowledge of such profound and intense education and training to achieve such nursing practice. It reminds me of when I served in the United States Navy, during Operation Desert Storm/Desert Shield, the intricacies of patient care management and supervision, which I performed. Having been educated and trained in the specifics of military medicine, to provide outstanding quality healthcare to the sailors and soldiers serving in the Persian Gulf Crisis. Notwithstanding, the outstanding and quality of healthcare provided to the families for every military service member by the readiness of all and every military medical teams. It will be as precedented as when nursing was first introduced to mankind. How awesome is that?

Yes, it will be awesome to become an integral member of such space healthcare team. As far-fetched as it sounds, there will be an undying need for professional licensed practical nurses, in the work place. Even if the work place is in space. I don't think, that there will be such a thing as intergalactic nursing practice, at least not in my lifetime. Though people are contemplating space travel to mars. As has been mentioned in the media, it would be a one-way trip. Which might have a medical team involved. What type of special medical and nursing education and training would it take, to be part of such U.S.A. Space Forces. It is too premature to forecast, at this time.

With the many medical and nursing practices that are currently in place, the need for professional licensed practical nursing, within the nursing infrastructure and healthcare organizations, will have its role, as professional licensed practical nursing evolves. There will always be a restructuring of healthcare practices at all medical and nursing platforms, along with all medical and nursing entities. From institutions that teach every facet of healthcare to every company and corporation that participate in support of quality nursing practices and patient/client care.

CHAPTER FIVE

DIVERSITY

Are You Talented?

THE ART OF licensed practical nursing is a talent. Talented or not is not the question. All art requires a particular kind of nurturing of talent, as does the licensed practical/vocational nursing. When a person takes the steps in becoming a practitioner of healthcare, like an artist chosen to master their craft, the talents of the art of nursing take on a refined role. How diverse the professionally licensed nurse becomes is interdependent on the availability of professional resources. The horizons of nursing are expansive. Therefore, in the panorama of healthcare, there are even television and movies that have nursing roles.

Paying close attention to details, there seems to be no distinction between the licensed practical nurse and the registered nurse in those performing roles. The licensed practical nurse appears to be overlooked, from the usage of primary theory to the extended applications of advanced medical and nursing theory, only with a greater responsibility. Almost like a ghost. Practicing healthcare, almost unseen. I have been in that position. From the implementing of doctors' orders, following up on medical/surgical treatments, procedures and administering medication and immunizations. Implementing orders delegated by a registered nurse integrates the licensed practical nurse in the professional performance of nursing. Professionally documenting in a plethora of various medical records, that is, medical records on paper and electronic medical documentations. Sequentially by way of several types of computerized devices. Such as, computer hardware, laptops, notepads and specially programed cellphones. Also, there is an array of software with inter-applicable, interchange as well as intra-communicable implementation, as the palettes by and on which, the professional application of medical and nursing terminology are applied.

Recognition may need to be redirected. Nurses on all levels have gone unrecognized in several areas for their contributions to mankind. Through delegation and scope of practice, notwithstanding, the boundaries and limitation, the professional licensed practical nurse performs and delivers, in the light of what appears to be no talent. Therefore, the instruments, by which the licensed nurse performs on, for describing what kind of nursing care has been implemented, become the palate. The palate of colors verbally expressed. The colors of medical and scientific terminology that produce professional and vivid expressions, designed specifically for the community of professional practitioners of healthcare. The scientific community may also have an advantage, by such presentations, since, the development of medical, surgical, therapeutic devices and pharmacological interventions are all codependent. How else, can the licensed nurse be able to deliver and contribute to the vision of the future of professional healthcare? If not for these devices, along with the contributions of the scientific community, it would be a great struggle.

Like a musician needs sheet music, to perform a musical composition, and the painter needs a canvas and brushes for the application of oil or acrylic colors, so does the professionally licensed nurse require specific tools and instruments, in order to deliver this fine art of practical nursing, on its platform of practice. The music has to be rhythmic, with the clarity of tone and a discernable melody. Imagine the healthcare teams and its components moving to the rhythm and flow, while providing care to its constituents.

Yes, there is a rhythm and a flow by which all members of the healthcare team move in concert. Which would be better known as the professional concerted effort. The timing, with which, healthcare is designed and set forth, in the provision of medical and nursing care, must be accurate and precise. Should there be a dysrhythmia of its rhythm and flow, there would be a disjointed disruption of what would be the concerted effort of nursing care and the healing process, like a wobble. That wobble would be more like a missing step or a misplaced step in the course of nursing practice. More like that of nursing negligence or malpractice. Therefore, the consistency of nursing practice makes for an exemplary performance of professional nursing.

Every area and clinical setting has a timing of its own, for example, at the emergency room, where treatments and procedures may need to be implemented in a rapid professional, efficient and effective manner. At the emergency department is where the utmost proficiency may become paramount to imperative nursing care. Not so fast. To be effective in producing the best of positive outcomes, all members of the healthcare and trauma teams need to be as thorough as possible. Obtaining such information as the mechanisms of trauma and illness. Obtaining a clear and accurate medical, surgical and mental health history as well as a social history. Including but not limited to persons involved and affected, when a patient/client experiences illness or a trauma. This type of rhythm may also apply, at the critical care clinical setting of nursing practice.

Transitioning from one area of practice to another area of practice, the professional nurse will need to adjust from tunes to melodies and from colors to shades of colors. The professional nurse cannot transition with a song and dance, but by being cognizant of the professional environment, the chain of the communication and the nursing care recipient. The recipient of practical nursing begins from administrative protocol to the end receiver, the customer. Between the two recipients are healthcare providers with specific and diverse practices.

The first healthcare recipient may be the employer who provides access to equipment and the customer client/patient, from onset of nursing care to the end care of professional nursing. The second recipient of professional nursing is the professional healthcare team and it's members. They may range from the security guards and front desk personnel, such as the receptionist clerk, to all the professional components of the healthcare team. Professional components may be the integrated departments that provide professional healthcare at a medical facility or community. With each specialty of healthcare, scientifically engaged, comes the area of practice relating to obtaining clear and concrete outcomes, for efficient and effective customer client/patient care. Therefore, with professional knowledge of clinical practice, the professional licensed practical nurse can or should include electrocardiographer, phlebotomy and wound care certifications or licenses to enhance their talents, within the team approach. This diversity of practice expedites the care and recovery of the client/patient receiving professional nursing care. Having an in depth knowledge of medical coding and billing may also be helpful to the professional licensed practical nurse which may facilitate the nursing care delivery process with more proficiency. Medical coding and billing is an administrative function and may not be complimentary to the facilitation of the professional nursing practice in the work place. Usually, the medical office assistant or a professional medical coder performs medical coding and billing, throughout the patient/client care process. Well-established foundation knowledge of the language and application of medical coding may increase proficiency and productivity.

To be articulate, in the performance of professional nursing, fine-tuning of the human senses may need some adjustments. An inappropriately tuned instrument will only produce unwelcomed noise. Whereas, the appropriately tuned instrument will produce the right sound, whether it is being played in a musical band or amongst the harmonious integration of an orchestra. At this juncture is where visiting some aspects from whence the education and training of practical nursing was introduced. Highlighting the natural human growth and development process, from the milestones of birth throughout the maturational process and into adulthood. Thereby, implementing this knowledge throughout the professional applications of practical nursing and evaluating outcomes, when faced with professional challenges.

The neonate is evaluated with the application of an APGAR score. (Appearance, how the neonate appears at the moment of birth. Pulse, is the neonatal heart beating rhythmically and strong or not. Grimace, What faces is the neonate making, if any. Activity, which denotes physical movements, such as, morrow reflex, grip and startle). Respiratory, are the lungs clear bilaterally and symmetrical. How does the neonate respond to its first social experience? Each and every sound, activity as well as the appearance of an individual provide a clinical description of the human experience. From the onset of our first breathe, the response of the first social experience to independence and mobility. Establishing the nature of crawling, walking through and up to the paces of running. The race to accomplish independence, development of agility and manual dexterity will form an individuals' identifying capabilities.

In the theater of medical and nursing practice, everyone has a role. Nature provides the script, the colors and the music. Just by when the neonate takes a hold of the pinky of the hand of the healthcare provider, be it the doctor, the midwife, the professional registered nurse or the licensed practical nurse, a message is sent and received. It is a dual message. The gripping of the pinky denotes, "thank you for being here for me". The prolonged holding if the pinky sending a message back to the newborn, "I will always be here for you". This is one of the most rewarding experiences the professional nurse could have. Priceless. With every aspect of the human being, from the color, texture, temperature and turgor of their skin, a narrative of ones life is captured. This narrative is complimented with the observations of the individual patient/client physical and mental growth and development, thereby, providing a detailed and picturesque expression of what level of healthcare may be needed for the provision and performance of professional nursing.

As is naturally known, there are five senses by which everyone fares through life. Actually, I will profess, there are six senses. There is the sense of touch, sight, smell, taste and the sense of sound. Everyone of the natural senses express the way a patient/client, subjectively, provides an initial point of patient/client health history to the professional nurse. By listening to the client/patient describe what they are experiencing, along with the professional observations of how the client/patient is providing such personal information, which will assist the professional nurse with interpreting, objectively, the sounds, colors, mobility and mental health status of the patient/client.

The scene is set. The players and performers are ready and in place. Hopefully, the script is clear and concrete. All that is about to happen is when, what type and level of healthcare will be implemented and how the patient/client will receive and respond to the implementation of nursing care by the professional nurse. Almost, like in a ballet, the application of an instrument, with the intent to reach a positive and outstanding goal, a certain level of professional versatility and dexterity may be required. Obtaining vital signs, specific specimens for testing and performing certain specific physical and mental examinations will provide the baseline norm of the patient/client. After all of the preliminary data is obtained, by the professional nurse, the data will then be conveyed to the professional audience of healthcare providers that will then interpret, objectively, as per each involved healthcare provider applies the professional interpretations. At this point, the stage is set. The curtain goes up and the goal for reaching an outstanding, positive and a satisfactory goal may be accomplished.

On the canvas, for implementing the colors, shades and nuances, lay the description of how the professional nurse may view the healthcare scenario. The palate of the application of such colors on the healthcare canvas, such as, that of the patient/client fabric of the skin. The skin can be described as appearing pink, black, brown, cyanotic blue, ecchymosis various shades of ecchymosis, from bluish to greenish or brownish; intact or having an abnormal appearance like abrasions, contusions, punctures, lacerations or burns. A variety of interpretations can be deduced just by the appearance of the skin. The iris, pupil, sclera and visual vascular aspects of the eyes present the appearance and superficial anatomical and physiological presentation of the eyes, as well. With every visual and auditory presentation of the patient/client state of health the professional nurse may implement refined talents through the process of performing nursing care.

The sixth sense is the gut feeling. The inner most feeling one interprets with. Which may help with conveying what the patient/client is experiencing. That gut feeling may usually be right on point, although, it may be better to exercise that interpretation on the side of caution. Which could be a sniffle, a whimper, the whine, a happy face, whether expressing a sweet, sour or bitter taste. Including the pursing of the lips. A cry could denote a discomfort, be it soft, loud or a scream. Including the universal facial expressions of crying, laughing, snickering, giggles and especially degree of pain or discomfort. The professional licensed practical nurse may apply such appearances and sound to the canvas and musical score, for professionally interpreting how the patient/clients are presenting themselves.

Healthcare providers rely on each other, therefore, the more talented the professional licensed practical nurse is, the more and greater possibilities that may arise. I profusely advocate that every professionally licensed nurse pursue professionally refining the practice of professional licensed nursing. Including and not limited to perusing all of the possibilities that can raise and broaden the horizons for the professional licensed practical nurse to be multi-talented, thereby, becoming multi-marketable. The possibilities can be endless, because the healthcare industry is ever changing and with change comes diversity.

From the classroom and clinical lab practice to the trenches of reality professional nursing practice, there are no actual boundaries in which the professional nurse may professionally perform at. So much diversity has existed, since the origins of practical nursing. Historically, going back as far as the Crimean War, from whence the great need of nurses became in demand to care for wounded soldiers. Throughout every battlefield, where war and crisis existed, especially with the affiliation of the United Stated of America, the professional licensed nurse performed patient/client care without reservation and with dignity. That same professionalism has been extended to civilians and their families throughout the century, on land, sea and air, globally and limitlessly.

Diversity has been practiced by the professional nurse, such as educators, from bedside patient teaching and at schools of professional continuing education. As professional educators, there has been, and always will exist, the need for professional nurses, to teach at the professional allied health levels, as well as, teaching at the high school levels. Motivating and inspiring students to become aspiring contributors to a world, where there is a great need of so much healthcare, throughout humanity. It may not need to be at the medical clinic, hospitals or nursing homes. Those newly found hopes and aspirations can also be brought into the local community and worldwide.

The licensed practical nurse may not be awarded any medals to wear or honors to hang on the wall, but it is not to say that medals and honor are privy. It is the talent and the professionalism that are the medals and honors of the professional nurse. The outstanding exemplary and positive contributions of professional licensed practical nursing contributing towards the positive health and welfare for all mankind. When the need arises for the professional licensed practical nurse to provide nursing on the practical level, there is no doubt that the talents, learned and refined will prevail. The healthcare profession does not fully, in fact, give recognition to the constituency of the professional nurse.

As defenders of life and comforters of the broken and as talented providers of healthcare; throughout the healing process of that mankind may be experiencing, the professionally licensed nurse, in sickness and in health, is a beacon of light for every client/patient passing through the rough roads and terrain of the world we all live on; that everyone who fares through, whether by land, sea or by air and without reservation, firm and ready. The professional nurse is a firm and integral pillar of nursing and healthcare that will be providing comfort professionally, for all humanity and the generations to come.

It has been said, that success is not achieved in thirty minutes nor in thirty days but by thirty years of experience and then some, in applying oneself to accomplish the service to humanity. (Inspired by an unknown author). Nurses at all levels, are the backbone of humanity and the world. Nurses are fearless. Nurses are not afraid of being at the forefront of the patient/client healthcare process. Nurses are brave and bold enough to confront any illness or disease that a patient/client may be overcome by and challenge that illness or disease throughout the brokenness being experience by the client/patient to the end. How beautiful and blessed are they? With the vast and diversified contributions to healthcare, the professional licensed practical nurse, faithfully and respectfully will continue to discharge the practice of healthcare as is deemed and absolutely.

CHAPTER SIX

FLEXIBILITY

Can You Move With It?

THE NURSING PROCESS is not a machine. No nurse is a rubber band. Though, all nurses are movers and shakers of the nursing process, the professional licensed practical nurse has a role to perform in the movements of nursing and healthcare. As an integral member of its moving parts, the professional licensed practical nurse, from being a nursing student to successfully becoming a professional licensed nurse, has demonstrated the ability to be flexible and diverse. Thereby, establishing the professionally licensed nurse as a well-oiled nursing and healthcare team member within the sum of its parts. As previously stated, nurses are the backbone of the health care delivery system and the world. Every nurse has been influenced, in becoming the best nurse that they can be, from the professional medical, surgical and nursing healthcare providers, to the professional providers of all healthcare entities and professions. By such influences, the licensed nurse would be flexible, versatile with a professional style of agility and ergonomically prepared. Motion and the nursing process go hand in hand. Whether it be, your hands or the hands of your team members. Hand in hand, the terminal objective, throughout the nursing process forges on. (Mano a Mano)

Therapeutically, the patient/client hands, also, have a significant role in the motions that move the performance of the nursing and healthcare process. This is where instruction, demonstrations and returned demonstrations go hand and hand. Shifting from nursing ease to medical ease and back to the professional communication is paramount to diversity and flexibility. This continual process is staple to efficient and effective nursing care by the professional nurse.

It would be nice, if we can all speak and comprehend all languages of the human race. It is virtually impossible that anyone could attain such talents, but nonetheless, the licensed nurse is an integral part of the mosaic of the professional healthcare delivery team. A professional nursing mosaic that is very rich in cultural, ethical entities and geo-demographic practices. Within these elements is where the dynamics and flexibility of the professional nurse are best expressed. Wherever the need for nursing care, the licensed nurse, having a well-rounded foundation, through professional practice, perform empathetically in such an integrated and diverse world.

Like every muscle, moving independently, there is a codependence and reliance on the central nervous system for such a coordinated effort. The brain receives a message by the stimulus of a nerve from, for example, either the skin or by any chemical, atom, molecule, cell tissue or any of the organs of the human body. A conveyed response to the stimuli may then be produced. Or not. The origins of the stimulus can be either internally produced or externally produced. This analogy is only a mild comparison of how the professional nurse performs. As an important integral member of the medical, nursing and professional healthcare community, the significant outcomes of the quality of professional nursing care performed and produced. With such coordination, the goals of providing outstanding, exemplary nursing care performed, assuring comfort throughout the healthcare and healing process can be attained. Therefore, the agility and dexterity of performing with a musical instrument a musical composition may analogous to the agility and dexterity by the artist painter producing the brush strokes, colors and shades of colors on the canvas.

Let's image another analogy, during a rush hour, at Grand Central Station, in New York City, where an innumerable amount of commuters are commuting to and from the city and various parts thereof. Coming and going to and from the tri-state and beyond. Transferring to and from motor vehicles, buses and trains. Traversing through the brash of commuters, vehicular traffic and the unforeseen delays. Then, imagine a change of shift, which occurs everyday, all week and all year long continuously 24/7/12 and 365. The transfer and the endorsement of client/patient care accompanied with a report and outcomes, at a non-stop pace with all hands on deck. All medical and nursing care performed, which includes a complete, accurate and true conveyance, through professional verbal reports with supporting documentation. Whereby, for each and every patient/client, having unique reasons, diagnosis, treatments, medications and procedures, a concise, accurate and concrete the reports are passed on. All this from the prior shifts the currently reporting shift and to the oncoming shift. Only to be re-endorsed again and again. (The shift report)

In the huddle of all members within the medical, nursing and healthcare professions, exists the reliance on the accuracy of each and every detailed aspect of the nursing reports. Like traffic moving through city streets, with flashing traffic lights that, whether red, green or yellow, every member of the medical, nursing and professional healthcare team must heed to every signal, sign or waving flag, in order to perform professionally and responsibly in a harmonious and smooth motion. The dexterity to perform any medical and professional nursing procedure will require specific education and training for producing outstanding, positive and quality nursing outcomes. The goal being to attain outstanding positive quality outcomes, as a result of applying professional licensed practical nursing theory without the production of untoward outcomes.

Time management in the nursing performance of the licensed nurse also, requires the reviewing of medical and nursing documentation; whether within computerized devices, manually documenting within the paper flow charts or within the pages of all professional medical documents. This review is time consuming and is mandatory and by law, required to be reviewed by each and every medical, nursing and healthcare professional who provide professional healthcare for the patient/client. Wherefore, it is paramount that the professionally licensed nurse be educated and trained in becoming familiar with the many variations and inter-related applications and methods by which the professional medical and nursing process is implemented, to become familiar with the computerized hardware, software and the mechanisms of such hardware and software that are implemented and documented into, also.

By the professional medical and nursing education and development process, the professional nurse may reduce the stresses that affect the performance of the delivery of professional nursing. Understanding the motions involved, through the professional dexterity of applying professional licensed practical nursing theory at the points of care for the patient/client, the professional licensed practical nurse, may also reduce the stressors accompanied throughout the professional medical and nursing process. Time and motion go hand in hand, throughout the professional medical nursing process. There are no short cuts. Every application of each and every medical procedure, treatment and device have been scientifically tried and tested before any professional nurse can implement such, medical and nursing procedure, treatment and medical equipment and device, for professional medical, nursing and therapeutic outcomes.

Therefore, timing is everything. The application of time management throughout the art of professional licensed practical nursing is essential. Like the musician producing a musical composition; the variations of timing and expression of the musical composition by the composer of such composition, has to be tightly composed. There may be a multi-scored musical composition with various movements throughout the musical composition. The musical composition may be composed for other members of a band or an orchestra. If the musical composition is mal-composed or mal-scored by the inappropriate placement of notation, timing and expression, the performance of the musical composition will be as clanging cymbals. The ballet will be as disjointed as trying to skip and hop at the same time. The audience will be dismayed at such an attempt to perform. Wherefore, timing is everything. Can you dance? Everyone is listening and watching. The clinical setting is your stage. Where and how the document is your canvas. So, perform professionally and responsibly. Mistakes may not be forgivable. The impact of mistakes can be a learning experience or a lifetime lesson.

From the start of a shift/tour at the healthcare facility to the end of a shift/tour, at the nurses station, the never ending passing of the patient/client nursing report is endorsed over to the relieving professional medical, nursing and allied healthcare providers. The continuum of the professional nursing and healthcare process is a twenty-four hour and seven days a week non-stop movement, which are the wheels by which each application of the professional nursing process must be well oiled. The wheels may be defined as the ultimate of being prepared in moving patient/client professional nursing care. The licensed practical nurse, therefore, becomes the vehicle by which to deliver practical nursing care. Through every degree of the nursing process, every patient/client will require individual attention.

Every professional healthcare practitioner must be relieved from medical and nursing practice at some point of every shift/tour. When taking a break, or needing to leave any healthcare setting a nursing report by the professional nurse, providing professional nursing care for a patient/client, which may be for an individual patient/client or several patient/clients, must provide a detailed nursing report to the medical doctor and/or professional registered nurse from whom an original medical and nursing report was transpired from, at the beginning of a shift/tour, for any reason. Upon returning from the break, be it a coffee/lunch break of the need to leave the healthcare setting, a report must be given back to the licensed nurse by the medical doctor and/or the registered nurse, of any new doctors orders, treatments or procedures rendered along with the outcomes. By the inter-communications of every professional healthcare providers, the delivery of professional nursing throughout the professional medical and nursing process continuum is maintained uninterrupted.

The motions and processes of professional nursing are determined by the diagnosis and treatments required for performing such nursing care. Every patient/client may have a diagnosis that will produce receiving unique quality nursing care. Every diagnosis will be unique to every aspect of a patient/clients health status. Therefore, every diagnosis being unique to every recipient of practical nursing, the time for treatments and procedure will have to be tapered and adjusted throughout the nursing and healthcare processes. It's almost like adjusting the time on a clock or a watch, within the microns of timing. Like the moving parts within the engine of a motor vehicle or a machine that allow each functional part to maintain a smooth rhythm in the motion of its moving parts. If any part of a clock or a watch, or even of a machine or motor if a motor vehicle were out of timing and rhythm, these mechanical devices would not function smoothly. More like, wobbly, lopsided and unbalanced nursing care.

Diverse and flexible, professional education and training development of the professional nurse can be attained, either horizontally or vertically. The horizontal professional developments, being the broadest, are more attainable. Throughout the scope of practice, the professional nurse may manage time, personal and professional responsibilities and obligations on a spectrum. Personal responsibilities and obligations are private to each professionally licensed nurse. From self and social development to environmental and global developments, there are several choices from which to choose from.

What forms the professional practice of the licensed practical nurse will depend on the private and personal influences, notwithstanding, the affects and such influences. Everyone is a world and even a universe that has been formed by the internal and external interpretations of achievements towards the attainments of positive and successful goals. One may even be expected to be glad and satisfied in achieving those goals. Like clay in the potters' hand, whole, becoming shaped and molded, it is the goal, throughout the professional practice of the licensed practical nurse, to become an outstanding work of art. A work of art developed, like a diamond in the rough; a work of art of the highest quality. A work of art produced to perform outstandingly professional. We are all human, but for reasons of a muddled world, the professional nurse is expected to preform flawlessly. That would be unrealistic but expected, nonetheless.

It will always be the responsibility and professional obligation, for keeping abreast of current and outdated modalities and practices, throughout the practices of professional nursing, therefore, to be proficient in practicing such changes and developments. Attending clinical in-service education and training workshops and seminars, at the workplace, would be the most economical, in terms of time and finance. Most places of professional nursing practice may facilitate clinical in-service and training, for staying abreast of medical and nursing applications of current methods and modalities for practical nursing. This type of in-service education and training can be excellent for in-house patient/client nursing practice, but is limited to and only for the institutions that provide in-house education and training. There may not be an acquisition of certification of such in- service, but necessary, nonetheless.

In order for the professional licensed nurse to, ultimately, be professionally informed and kept current of changes and practices of licensed nursing, attending professional workshops and seminars offered by licensed organizations will be helpful. In certain clinical nursing facilities, may even be mandatory. Through at length and in depth, continuing professional education and training, for the attainment of professional certification of a specialty practice: be it as a phlebotomist or medical research specialist, attending a specialty class at an institution of higher education may be the best way to go.

It's like putting oil or hydraulic fluid to certain points of professional nursing practice. Moving right along, through the acquisition of specialized professional education and training, the licensed nurse may become as flexible and diverse and may be deemed necessary. Performing with the fluidity of flawless professional licensed practical nurse upgrading, may also prevent such cramping, stunting and the stiffness of the methods and motions for implementing advanced licensed practical nursing, treatments and procedures; complimented by continued professional education and training of such professional enhancements, for recertification.

The demand for professional flexibility and adaptability of the professional licensed practical nurse with the potential of acclimating in a variety of diverse medical and professional licensed practical nursing practice is great. Being Diverse, fluidly flexible and adaptable are desirable attributes of the professional licensed practical nurse. It can be overwhelming, in the general or specialty implementations of practical nursing, to challenge such diversity in the practice of any level of professional nursing. Therefore, it is strongly advisable to manage time and stress in ones personal and professional aspects of the professional nurse. Some of the strongest and most desirable attributes of the professionally licensed nurse are being current, diverse, flexible and adaptable, when preforming professional nursing functions. The faithful and professional dispensing of nursing having the utmost respect of patient/client, throughout the process of professional nursing are essential.

It would seem effortless, in the provision of professional nursing, but in fact, a great amount of effort is exercised in the performance of professional nursing patient/client care. By such great, implemented effort, exemplary and outstanding quality outcomes of patient/client care are attained. Inclusively, throughout the performance of licensed practical nursing, the safety and protection and reassurance of each and every patient/client is always of great concern. It is not to imply that the professional nurse bear arms for the protection of the patient/client, but by the professional implementation of specific laws, rules, regulations, policies and procedures, throughout the professional nursing process, patient/client privacy is maintained.

It is by the fluidity of professional healthcare communications, which facilitate the adaptability, and the diverse flexibility of the professional nurse, in practice. By the stretch of such communications, medical, nursing and professional providers of healthcare are able to reach as far as is possibly imaginable, the delivery, performance, well being and monitoring of medical and professional licensed nursing provide for the patient/client. Inclusively, even for the astronauts in outer space. Wow. Communicating at the speed of light and the speed of sound. That is fast. Well, not so fast now. Let's take into account that it would actually take an exceptionally and scientifically professionally educated and trained team of professional healthcare providers to deliver and monitor such a fine level of healthcare. As scientific as healthcare may be, the professionally licensed nurse, at its finest scope of practice, may also be a participant of such astronomical nursing care. This is how, through the thoroughness of pre-preparation for spaces flight, leaving earth, and the post care from the return of space flight back to earth. Therefore, before anyone may be flown into space, specific data sets, from vital signs and human body specimens to behavioral data, may be ascertained with the participating assistance of the professional nurse.

Whether at the military or at a NASA facility for advanced professional healthcare surveillances and monitoring, the status of health of a person being flown into space will necessitate health monitoring and documentation. It is what happens at space school training. Including every participant, from the scientific community of space engineers, medical and nursing professionals at the earth monitoring space centers. Especially, for diagnostic and prognosticating evaluations, like that of the HEDIS medical records review, only much more intense and scientifically detailed. And that is just the tip of the iceberg. What lies ahead in the future is yet to be explored; this just may be the pivotal point for licensed nursing. After all, an astronaut must pass through the halls of military medical facilities, be examined to be medically qualified, to be transported into outer space. There, at the military medical and healthcare facilities, is where the professionally licensed nurse is an integral member of such a refined and detailed professional healthcare team.

To think that such diversity of professional practical nursing emerged from military education and training and military medical licensed practical nursing is the most refined and rigid of any kind of practical nursing. Civilian education and training of the practical nurse is just basic to the practice of nursing taught at the civilian community level. It is hoped, that at any level of nursing, the professional licensed practical nurse provide exceptional and outstanding professional nursing care to its recipient patient/client for such exceptional, outstanding, exemplary quality and positive outcomes, not for the money.

Health Evaluation Data and Implementation Sets (HEDIS) are approximately ninety-one healthcare data sets measures and counting. Every year the HEDIS evaluation process changes, depending on specific developments in healthcare. Although HEDIS may not be implemented at prisons and military installations, the benefits for civilian and community healthcare evaluation of the delivery of healthcare is necessary. With the implementation of the HEDIS reviews and the implementation of the Nursing Counsel of Quality Assessments (NCQA), the approach for the professional healthcare of the patient/client may demonstrate a level of professional healthcare and accountability of such care. There too, is where the professionally licensed nurse is a participant and an integral member of the HEDIS teams. Through the collection of such healthcare data sets the quality, dynamics and consistency of professional healthcare may be reviewed and evaluated. These healthcare data sets include the medical coding and review of diagnosis, treatments, procedures, diagnostic procedures for diagnostic and therapeutic treatment and prognosis of the patient/client. (See The International Diagnostics Codes (ICD9 or higher) manual at your place or institution of professional medical and nursing practice) An in depth knowledge by professional education and training in medical coding may be required, for the application and implementation of medical records review and abstraction.

There are several types of professional medical and nursing organizations by which professional medical and nursing practices are evaluated. These evaluations may be local, state, national an international evaluations for the best interest of quality professional healthcare of every human being. From the prenatal stages and throughout the lifespan of every individual patient/client, the normal childhood milestones of human growth and development throughout adolescence and adulthood including the illnesses and diseases that may be acquired and challenged throughout the lifespan of the patient/client.

In essence, HEDIS is the surveillance and monitoring, through evaluation, of the health status, from conception to birth and up to end of life for the prevention and treatment of illness and disease. Through HEDIS reviews is where the integration of every provider of professional healthcare may have professional healthcare input that may affect the professional healthcare and health maintenance of the patient/client. Inclusively, the professional licensed practical nurse can be an integral member of the HEDIS medical records reviews teams. The HEDIS medical records review professional licensed practical nurse may include working remotely from home or may need to travel to and from the clinical setting; which may be at a doctor's offices, medical clinics, hospitals or nursing homes. Depending on the type of medical records review to be performed. Every medical facility may have its own type of computer hardware and software that is implemented for a chosen type medical style and medical practice. There may be the paper medical records review, for HEDIS and other medical abstraction. Now that is diversity and flexibility of professionally licensed nursing. Medical records reviews and abstraction may occur monthly, quarterly, seasonally annually or as needed, depending on the healthcare organization and its requisites. Because of ongoing changes, adjustments and additions to the professional healthcare delivery process, several adjustments are required for an accurate medical records review and abstractions, when these changes occur. There may be upgrades or new advances in professional medical and healthcare practices.

Medical records reviews are not limited to the healthcare workplace. Medical records reviews may be performed by the professionally licensed nurse at law offices for use as confirmation of evidence in litigation. This type of medical legal record review may be presented in the litigation of personal injury, products liability and medical malpractice cases, et al. These medical legal records reviews require specific education and training of the legal language applied to each individual lawsuit involved. There are specific rules of law and regulations for which a case must be of merit. There is also, becoming familiar with how and when a case is filed in the jurisdictional courts.

Being that there are over two hundred plus legal specialties of the practice of law, the dynamics of every legal application of law, by the representing attorney or law firm, will require certain legal authorization for the acquisition, review and applications of such medical records. Every release of medical information by the litigant will need to be notarized and filed, a lengthy and legal process at that. There are certain procedures and for continuance of a medical legal case for legal filing and up to the verdict of such case. Therefore, the professional licensed nurse may be a participant of many legal aspects of professional organizations. (See Legal Rules and Regulations in your state).

Becoming an allied health educator has unique challenges, for the professional nurse, when choosing to be an instructor and teacher of the allied health professions. These are great challenges. Developing a well-rounded foundation of human growth and development requires a certain level of professional immersion, by which to understand, as professionally as possible, as much of every student/candidate as possible. Students of professional healthcare education and training are from a varied mosaic of countries, cultures and traditions. Therefore, a professional and mature degree of the applications for teaching and instruction are a departure from the bedside and clinical patient/client teaching, from the point of care process, and is paramount when applied at the classroom and lab practice teaching and instructional points of professional education and training.

The teaching and instructional dynamics may range from teaching theory, practice and even experiential. How the student of professional allied healthcare is educated, taught and trained is crucial for professional healthcare practice. Facets that affect the delivery of the didactic and academics include but are not limited to the educator and instructor of professional allied heath education being aware and respectful of such a mosaic of students.

As a professionally licensed nurse, I have been exceptionally privileged and blessed, whereby, being grandfathered into the academia of the halls of professional allied health as professionally licensed private school teacher. In 1985, there was a call, by The University of The State of New York for competent nurses assistant instructors. Having always kept up with the changes in the performance of professional nursing, I took the leap of faith, and I applied for the challenge of becoming an instructor of the allied health professions. It is an experience that I will never forget; to teach an intense course of three hundred hours for certifying nurses assistants. At this juncture, being responsible for classroom theory and classroom lab instruction and practice.

While teaching the certified nurses assistant course, I was encouraged to enhance my teaching skills. I then enrolled in classes of electrocardiography, phlebotomy and various levels of medical office assistants. From frontline clerical medical office assistants, certified clinical medical assistants to administrative medical assistants with variations in medical coding and billing. I took the plunge. I became professionally licensed, by The University of the State of New York, in addition to being licensed to teach certified nurses assistants, I became licensed to teach, certified electrocardiograph technicians, certified phlebotomy technicians, and every level of medical office assistants.

By applying myself, through the professional enhancements in my career, I have been able to apply such theory for advanced practice in professional practical nursing. This specialized education and training of the professional allied health fields came together when I was referred to a United States Navy Recruiter. On December 1988, after having my professional nursing license and professional allied health licenses reviewed by the United States Navy, I was enlisted in the United States Naval Medical Corps. While having been trained for military service, I was recommended to become an instructor of military medicine for which I attended special classes in military medicine for the Persian Gulf Crisis. As a result of such specialized training, I trained independent duty corpsman in the specialized treatments and care of military personnel mobilized to and from the theater of war. It was as intense as being in the battlefield. I got medals and accolades too. It was an honor serving my country, citizens and mankind.

However, from professional developments, by professional healthcare education and training, there are several variations of practice as a professionally licensed nurse. Actually, there may be no end, of what the professional nurse can practice. There are boundaries and limitations, though. Within the realms of mental health and physical health education and training there are also the environmental aspects, which may affect the outcomes of professional nursing practice.

The following methods of applying practices in nursing need being mindful of. First sight nursing practice, which is primarily based on what is observed of the patient/client. Odiferous nursing practice, which influence the environmental and psychological response by professionals and persons within the proximity of odor presented by affected individuals. Taste bud nursing, an analogy, expressing the affects a nursing situation is presented. Whether tastefully presented or something presented in bad taste. Nursing by sound. Infers to what is heard by the medical and nursing professionals, such as, type of cry, moan, groan and volume of such sounds. In particular, tactile nursing, which is to touch and feel or not to touch and define. And finally gut nursing. How the gut feeling may determine or form a belief and response.

CHAPTER SEVEN

TAKING CHARGE

Can You Handle It?

WITH THE LATIN term "carpe-diem" we take the day in hand and hold on to the day. So much occurs throughout the day, which holds the seconds, minutes and the hours, twenty-four hours a day. From sun up through sundown, seven days a week, three hundred and sixty five days a year. The world is ever changing and only the zeitgeist holds the next moment in time, full with suspense and surprises. To be prepared, confident, flexible and diverse, the licensed practical nursing takes on the lessons of professionalism, thereby, becoming ready to take charge or not. Every person is a world in the constellation of events. The professionally licensed nurse, in the drivers' seat or pilots seat, will need to be prepared and ready for the bumpy roads or the turbulence and make a smooth landing. Like a pilot of plane, in flight, flying through the currents of air. Making the turbulent air feel like a breeze in the wind. Like the captain of the ship, sailing on choppy seas, through swells, gale force winds, severe currents and the ebbs of tides, navigating by way of the North Star, producing a smooth sailing. Like being at the wheel of an all terrain vehicle, traversing roads, with its twists and turns. Roads that may not have signs or traffic lights for crossing intersections safely. Who would even imagine, getting through such unknowns.

The day begins with the report of past, present and current events. Specific events that occur in the life and times of a person, events and incidences that shape the entire health and well being of a persons' lifestyle. Events that affect not just the person faring the world, also, the people, family, friends and significant others including their pets, notwithstanding the workplace other environments where individuals for which human interactions are crucial for surviving what may produce chaos. The busyness of home and thoroughfare's, community and world events, with sunny, calm and pleasing days, no one can predict what nature, human nature and the nature of things have in store, or may present. So much unpredictability, and the professional licensed practical nurse is like the captain of a vessel faring through. It is written in the scriptures, God will not place such burdens on anyone incapable.

On the continuum of professional licensed practical nursing, through which the safe, efficient and affective delivery of prudent nursing care occurs, exist the depiction and measure of professional licensed practical nursing. How tight or loose of a grip on the practice, as a professional licensed practical nurse, one may have, may determine the outcomes of that carpe diem. While holding on to the reigns of practicing, this art of practical nursing, do not hold the reigns too loosely, not even for a moment. For it is by distraction, misattribution and misinterpretation of events that the plane may fall, the ship may sink and the all terrain vehicle may be lost. The navigational map by which the professional licensed practical nurse has been set a course on will depend on how well prepared and plotted it is. Following every, and all of the directions of the well-plotted map will guide the professional nurse in traversing through the realm of healthcare. Thereby, performing professionally, efficiently and effectively the medical and nursing care warranted for each and every patient/client.

All things considered, becoming knowledgeable and confident, in the practice of professionally licensed nursing will be appreciated. The certainty of being professionally prepared and proficient with performing procedures and treatments, ordered by a licensed medical doctor or delegated by the registered nurse, will also determine the outcomes of professional licensed practical nursing. In the patient/client medical records is where the navigational map is plotted. Directions, beacons, outcomes are flagged throughout the patient/client medical records. Also known as "The Map. Every provider of professional healthcare will have input of which type and level of professional healthcare should be administered and performed.

There are several variations of professional medical doctors offices, medical clinics, hospitals, nursing homes and rehabilitation facilities where the practice of professional nursing is performed. While being a student of practical nursing, are commonly known as clinical areas of healthcare practice. But when actually preforming as the professionally licensed nurse, may be known, roughly, as the trenches. Why, the trenches? Because, in reality, so much is going on; on so many different and diverse levels, that, to produce the most positive and outstanding of outcomes, will require wearing the armor of professional nursing, to attain the highest possible quality of positive and outstanding practical nursing outcomes. The armor for the performance of professional practical nursing cannot be manufactured. That specific armor is earned and acquired by strictly adhering to the professional code of ethics required for the licensed nurse. That armor is to be worn at all times. Whether at home, civilian environments, at the clinical areas of practice and in the trenches of the battlefields, where it is of critical and of the utmost crucial moments. Never dropping or letting go of the armor that protects and defends the patient/client and especially yourself and fellow professional healthcare practitioners, in the performance and delivery of patient/client healthcare.

Although, by the direction of the licensed medical doctor, the endorsement for medical and nursing care may be delegated by licensed professional registered nurse to the licensed practical nurse, who then may delegate, to some degree, the nursing care for a patient/client, to the certified nurses assistant, the patient care technician, the patient personal care aide or to the home health aide. Whereby, the collection of patient/client healthcare data is transmitted, whether by paper or digital computer devices, from the latter healthcare provider through the ranks up to the former delegator of such medical and nursing care. Within the realms of professional nursing practices, there are nurse managers, nursing supervisors and various other levels of professional nursing practices; that may direct and oversee the delivery, performance and outcomes on the continuum of professional healthcare and nursing.

Like the corpsman and the medic, in the battlefield in the theater of war, is sovereign and independent, so is the licensed nurse, in the field of healthcare and professional nursing. Therefore, from where, to whom and how nursing care is delegated and performed as well as by whom is of paramount responsibility for the nursing outcomes of the patient/client. The patient/client will return to their home, community for recovery and rest and hopefully display and/or express the outcomes of such patient/client medical and/or nursing care.

Rewind. From the origins of practical nursing, in the frontline, for the urgent and imperative need of proficient medical, surgical nursing care, before there were any nurses or persons that could or would provide any degree of nursing care. Before there were any sets of qualifications that anyone could attain such recognition to perform any medical, nursing procedures and nursing treatments, there were people who genuinely had a propensity for the healthcare of the injured, the infirmed throughout the course of their lives. There was no time to think of what to do or even how to perform such needed nursing care. Something needed and had to be done. This is another way of being in the trenches of healthcare. It could have been anyone, anywhere and by any and all means possible. Such as the Good Samaritan whom at a roadside came across an injured person, and without prejudice or reservation, cared for this individual and nursed his wounds. With only empathy and the genuine desire to care for an injured and suffering individual,

The Good Samaritan stopped from being on his own journey to provide such care. That is the true love and desire performed and displayed by a caring person for a complete stranger of whereabouts unknown.

In the theater of war and crisis, came the medic and corpsman of which the practical nurse has its origin. The term practical denotes the actual performance of hands on applications of treatments and procedures relevant and significantly required, for the comfort, dignity and healing of an affected person. Specifically, the soldiers and sailors, that during times of war and crisis, before, at and after returning for battle, were all, in need of medical and nursing care. One could only, and maybe not even, fathom what actually occurred, in those times, on the battlefield, for that matter, at sea, on land or even in the air.

From the battlefields of the Crimean War, World War I, World War II, The Korean War, The Vietnam Crisis War, The Persian Gulf Crisis and every United States Military Expedition, the proliferation and progression of professional licensed practical nursing have come a long way. Inclusively, surviving the depression of the 1920's and a plethora of recessions. The professionally licensed nurse has contributed incredibly, great and by professional performance contributions to the delivery and implementation of healthcare and nursing. A great community of nurses, from Phoebe, Florence Nightingale, Clara Barton, Military and civilian nurses have performed and dispensed some of the greatest humanitarian contributions of professional medical and nursing healthcare for the cumulative and counting best interest, without prejudice or reservations, for mankind and the world.

In such theaters of war or moments of crisis, is truly where the confident and professional care of soldiers, sailors and people take charge. Boldly and courageously doing the very and optimal best in providing and performing life saving professional medical and nursing treatments and procedures for the military service men and women, so that they may return home safely. Not just for military service men and women but to people of totally and completely from other countries, towns, and communities of various cultures, customs and traditions, without prejudice or reservation. Who had time for prejudice or reservations? Sometimes immediate and the most imperative and paramount urgency had to be done, without question. Along with an immeasurable support of the loyal faithfulness and totality of the armed forces to perform the lifesaving of all at risk accomplished and done.

Fast forward, to the 21st century. With the proliferation of modern healthcare monitoring, providers of quality professional medical and nursing implementations, all professionally licensed nurses and the entire healthcare industry are, by law, required to be continually upgrading, updating and continually in communication throughout healthcare systems. Almost, in perpetuity while living and practicing within the realms of professional nursing. Whereby, at this juncture, are deemed professionally responsible and accountable for, no matter what, where or when, of being professionally in charge of the discharge, dispensing, performance and implementation of professional medical and nursing treatments, procedures and protocols including and not limited to the professional allied health ancillary personnel.

While serving in The United States of America Armed Forces, is where I was educated and trained, specifically, in the most special and intricate of medical and nursing treatments and procedures protocols known to man. The civilian schools of medical and nursing education and training could not even come close to teaching and learning of what truly goes on, within the whole world of professional medical and nursing care for all humanity and then some, especially at the levels of military medicine and nursing. There are so many aspects from atomic, molecular, cytological, histological, organic, systemic, entomologic, from reptile all the way through mammalian life that affect the professional performance and delivery of professional licensed nurse. Inclusive are the elemental, chemical and environmental influences, of the performance and delivery of professional licensed nursing.

For the army medic and the naval corpsman to be prepared and ready and take on the heaviest of patient/clients, the highest degree of dignity, respect and professionalism must be exercised. The specific and special combat operations within the realms of military medicine and nursing care, casualties of war and the traumas that the soldiers and sailors may experience, special education and training, that is, frontline and combat medical practice, become of the utmost importance. The combat medic and combat corpsman will always be in the gravest of danger. No scenario, where casualties of war exist is safe. The combat medic and combat corpsman including with the assistance of all military servicemen and women, create, manage and perform life saving treatments and procedures, on the spot. Taking charge of the tragic moment and preform all necessary treatments and procedures to soldiers, sailors and civilians affected in the theater of war. Throughout the theater of war, that is, anywhere in the world, be it on the shore and on land, at sea and any waterways, as in the deep sea in and on a submarine and in the air, healthcare is performed.

These are the true trenches. On land, in a fox hole, in front of or behind bushes and trees; in front of or behind rocks, on sand and sand dunes, inside and around caves, inside or behind the walls of buildings, hospitals, clinics, homes, tents and huts on any street highway or byway, on and/or inside boats, ships and submarines. Including on or inside of tanks, Humvees, jeeps and battlefield ambulances but not limited to helicopters, airplanes and jets, on or in any vehicle for rescuing and transporting, casualties, victims, military servicemen, especially medics and corpsman. Including the rescue and transport of military service dogs and animals. Including any and all methods for transporting whomever and whatever necessary, even by horse and buggy. For all that exists in the trenches, are specific policies and procedures, relevant at the theaters of war and crisis.

The treatments and procedures are initiated with a rapid assessment of every mechanism of trauma, life threat assessments and the rapid stabilization, by the application of specific treatments and procedures. In warfare, treatments and procedures include the stabilization of bleeding and hemorrhage, prevention of shock, administration of medication, such as, morphine sulfate injection and battlefield surgery. In the theater of war, there are no medical doctors or surgeons. Military medical doctor's and surgeons are at the mobile hospital, on land or shores, where casualties are received for treatments and procedures including emergency medical and surgical procedures. The combat medic and combat corpsman are the extensions of the medical doctors and surgeons. Performing immediate medical and surgical diagnostics. Dispensing and administering whatever medications, by whatever method necessary, that is, oral, sublingual, topical, subcutaneous, intradermal, intravenous and intramuscular injection. Including initiating an intravenous infusion line for infusing parenteral fluids and medication.

Assessing thoroughly, everything, while continuously taking in to account every-and all wartime activity on the battlefield. Guns firing, bullets flying, bombs exploding incoming rocket and missile fire. Including amphibious traffic, ships waiting for receiving casualties, while sending troops to the battlefield, including assessing and evaluating simultaneously, all of the chaos on and off the battlefield. All while preparing casualties of war, with life threatening injuries and trauma, as a result of all the chaos on and within the theater of war. So much, so fast and having only a micron of time for which to act, perform, stabilize, treat and transport such casualties of war as rapid and as safe as possible. Including the reassuring of the casualty/patient throughout their traumatic experience. Application of trauma bandages and trauma dressings for punctures, lacerations from projectiles and shrapnel. Application of special abdominal lap pad dressings after a casualty experiences abdominal evisceration, also. A professional and timely response for saving lives is performed.

The independent combat medics and the independent duty corpsman perform specific medical and surgical procedures, within the theater of war and crisis. Therefore, an intense education and training of medicine and surgery, practiced at actual hospital and clinical settings by military medical doctor's and military surgeons of several military medical and surgical specialties. Then and only then, within such military medical and surgical teaching institutions, will the combat medic, independent duty combat corpsman, including the military clinical hospital medic and hospital corpsman acquire such specialized medical and surgical education and training. From amputations, de-gloving and evulsions, the medical and surgical combat medic and combat corpsman will be specifically and specially educated and trained to perform. Taking charge by efficiently and effectively handling medical and surgical emergencies, by all means necessary, is how an outstanding, exemplary positive and quality goal must be accomplished. Especially, when critical life saving timing is of essence.

Whether in the civilian environment of professional medical and nursing practice or at the theater of war and crisis, whereby, being in complete charge and autonomous, as well as, being professionally cognizant of what it truly means to be in charge of any situation, a certain degree of professional readiness is paramount by the professional licensed practical nurse. Similarly, a professional nursing report of every client/patient must be endorsed accurately and without equivocation. This report will occur at every clinical medical and nursing unit by the licensed nurse, to which such report was endorsed by. Whether by the licensed medical doctor, professional registered nurse, another licensed nurse, the certified medical assistant or a duly responsible professional healthcare provider.

The professionally endorsed nursing report, is then, evaluated by the professionally licensed nurse, on the prioritization and implementation of professional medical and nursing treatment's and procedures. After such evaluations are completed, the delegation of patient/client care may be endorsed and assigned by the professionally licensed nurse, to the certified nurses assistant, patient care technician, nurse technician, according to the education and training, including, clinical experience of such ancillary personnel.

There may be a similarity, when professional agility and dexterity are simultaneously implemented, throughout professional patient/client nursing care, within civilian and military environment's. It would appear, almost magically, when the simultaneous implementation of theory and practice produced by the applications in treatments and procedures, performed well, is where true tender-loving-care lives. The seamless and fluid nursing process would accomplish such a magical experience, "The flower cannot grow by packing the soil too tightly, only by the tender planting of the seed".

Shifting through civilian licensed nursing practice is where the implementation of practical nursing treatments and procedures are usually implemented, for the patient/client experiencing trauma, illness or disease. A traumatic incident may be experienced on a civilian street, client/patients home, community recreation area, school or civilian workplace. Then and only then, at such civilian environments, may the professionally licensed nurse provide life saving and or life stabilizing procedures independently, until the proper 911 personnel arrive. Independent practice by the professionally licensed nurse may also be implemented, when there is a local or national act of war and terrorism occurs, if appropriately educated, trained and mobilized. Such as, the chaotic and tragic events of the 9-11-01, World Trade Center attacks at Ground Zero and vicinity, The Pentagon and on Flight 163. Continued search and rescue operations would, then, be performed by appropriate national incident emergency and appropriate assigned national, federal, state and local emergency response personnel. Professionally licensed medical and nursing healthcare providers will, therefore, be on standby for mobilization, as ordered by the appropriate government offices.

On this anecdote, I was mobilized by a, FEMA registry for nurse's agency for the support of all mobilized military, fire fighter, enforcement and rescue personnel. My assignment was at the Bellevue Hospital and the World Trade Center Ground Zero. Due to my specialized military education and training on war and crisis of mass trauma victims and medical life threat treatment and stabilization, I was charged with the training of supporting medical and nursing personnel for the receiving and treating of surviving casualty victims. It was a sight to see the living casualty victims of the World Trade Center arrive at the Bellevue Hospital Center Emergency Department. They were stunned and in shock by the World Trade Center events. Special and empathetic emotional support was immediately implemented.

At this level and degree of being a first responder, there are local police, port authority police, state police, and local and city firefighter personnel along with an array of special operations and Federal Emergency Management Administration (FEMA) personnel. At such a tragic and chaotic incident, the most urgent and imperative response is the implementation of rescuing and stabilization of the surviving victims of such a chaotic, tragic and traumatizing incident. As was experienced, all levels, from national, military, federal, state, city and local professional agencies will be mobilized. Such an impact on The United States of America, which created a ripple affect, both nationally and internationally, have sent the message to every citizen, in The United States of America and abroad. The highest degree of professional medical and nursing must be actualized. Whereby, raising the bar on national, state, city and local professional licensed medical and nursing practitioners for such emergent events. Including all allied health and civilian persons, businesses, corporations and companies heretofore.

There is no civilian professional provider of healthcare services or academic schools that provide no academic military professional medical and nursing education or training. No tour of military education and training, not on a warship, a carrier, boat, submarine, airplane, jet, helicopter military installation, desert or shore, with the exception of being affiliated with The Veterans Administration hospitals and clinics. (See Veterans Administration of the United Stats of America) No civilian military wartime, tragedy, or battlefield education and training and exercise on such scenarios are offered.

Surviving and graduating such rigid military medical and nursing education and training exercises to be certified, for the performance of medical and nursing treatment and surgical procedures, requires a strong, mature, and an accomplished well rounded and disciplined foundations on war and crisis. For immediate, rapid, thorough assessment, psychological, physiological and environmental affects on war and crisis which has affected servicemen and civilians. Inclusive, a healthy psychological and physiological state of health, to be capable of taking charge, for the safety of self, and the protection and safety of fellow servicemen and civilians. The professionally licensed nurse, performing and implementing such immediate, emergent and imperative nursing practice, performs with the concerted efforts of all first responder personnel. The licensed nurse must be capable and able to adapt and acclimate in and at the most chaotic, tragic conditions and environments.

I would, therefore, recommend for my civilian professional licensed nurses and cohorts, in the professional provision of healthcare, to enlist in any of the United States Armed Forces as a reservist or full active duty. The United States of America needs exceptionally educated and trained professional medical and nursing providers as well as allied health personnel. Because no one will ever know when such tragedy may occur, whether on a small scale or on a more pronounced scale. Professional licensed practical nursing readiness is an outstanding and exemplary professional quality.

On a softer note, by which casualties of war and crisis are received, whether at a trauma facility on land, sea or on air, the most empathetic of the most rigid but caring with tender loving care (TLC) need be provided. Soldiers, Sailors and all military personnel, who have experienced traumatic and incapacitating tragedy, in the battlefield and theater of war, incur deeper and unseen non-visual wounds; both, physiological and psychological as well as environmental combined, long term. Notwithstanding, the post-traumatic affects of specific treatments and procedures, implemented on the battlefield. With the most caring and genuine implementation of TLC for not only the servicemen, their families, loved ones and significant others; it is hoped, beyond unimaginable hope, civilian casualties inclusively, that all professional providers of medical and nursing interventions and the care thereof, on every level, produce the highest, most outstanding, exemplary and positive quality of care. The truest, competently outstanding, exceptional of professional providers of healthcare are born there.

Whereas, on a more civilian note, the continuity of quality professionally licensed nursing practice, having been, and implemented, throughout civilian healthcare continuum, have supported every sector of professional medical and nursing throughout war and crisis, to the well, the affected and the infirm. Anyone can become a victim of acts of terrorism. The ripple affects and repercussive affects can be as traumatic as what has been incurred from war and crisis. Nonetheless, upon the reception of such traumatized persons, the same level of dignified, most highest outstanding, urgent and imperative, exemplary quality of care is merited, respectfully and rightfully so. Regardless of who is affected, by such traumatic experience, the professional licensed nurse will perform and implement any and all inclusive professional medical and nursing treatments and procedures, as required by law, without prejudice or reservation. Whereby, attaining the highest and outstanding, exemplary, without equivocation of positive outcomes. The ultimate goal is to provide and meet the highest outstanding quality of life for patient/client comfort and satisfaction with respect and dignity for all mankind. Inclusively, providing professional licensed practical nursing care for infants, children and adults in foster care and rehabilitative pediatrics.

When a child or adult is separated from the nurturing person they know, it can be quite traumatizing. Not as when going to school for the first time, or, by having to get on a school bus for the first time. The severing of such child/children and parent(s) bond is quite the traumatic experience. The bond developed by parent/caregiver and child is like the strongest link of a chain, hard to break. Everyone is a stranger out of the infant and child comfort zone. The professionally licensed nurse is no exception, when a child experiences such separation. Since the infant child has no vocabulary, short of mama, and that would the universal expression by infants from multitudes of cultures, and countries internationally, or the facial expressions that universally provide infant communications, there is the confused look displaying, "who or what are you"? or the look of acceptance expressing "OK treat me nice and I won't cry". "I could cry pretty loud, you know". The coos and babbles that only an infant understands. The sad look, the look that expresses "I am not feeling up to what is making me feel bad", the happy and satisfied facial expressions. To mention a few of the vast and universal expressions, thereby, display of facial and non-verbal communications expression. It is paramount to become familiar with each child's level and form of communication, individually. Children have the sixth sense of gut feeling. Every infant child is in charge if himself. And they will let everyone know about it.

The nursing care of the infant and child may be performed at several places, including the home. There are various hospitals at which the professionally licensed nurse may provide practical nursing care, such as, the general or community hospital on a general pediatric unit. At such general pediatric unit, there may be infants and children that may have experienced episodes of an illness, which require professional healthcare stabilization and monitoring. Or may need specific treatments or procedures that can only be performed at a hospital within a medically controlled environment. At an emergency room department, where urgent and immediate nursing care may need to be performed, due to possible or life threating trauma or illness. Especially when an infant or child is brought to the emergency department by ambulance, after being primarily stabilized by professionally certified emergency medical technicians.

There are specialty hospitals where the infant child may have been born with a congenital handicap or disability. Some infants and children may have multiple handicaps and multiple disabilities. To meet the nursing needs of such infants and children, who have such varying degrees of a handicaps or disabilities, the professionally licensed nurse will need to be well versed, educated and professionally mature to perform specialty professional nursing at such specialty healthcare facilities. To provide the most empathetic and most sensitive of patient/client care, under the most sensitive and stressful environments and conditions; it is paramount that a mature, skillful and professional demeanor, be had by the professionally licensed nurse. Especially when an eminent end of life moment occurs. Every professional medical and nursing staff as well as all personnel providing professional care and attention is affected, to some degree, in one way or another. At this juncture, every professional medical and nursing provider, including all ancillary personnel may provide emotional support for the entire team. Inclusive of that support are the families, friends and significant persons and pets.

Children in foster care experience traumatic injury much different than the child at their own homes. The question of "what will happen to me now" may arise. Due to so much uncertainty by the child and the unpredictability the child is faced with. To dissipate and defuse such uncertainty that that child in foster care is experiencing, reassuring the foster child will be paramount for the attainment of the compliancy of the child. The foster child should be encouraged to participate in the healthcare treatment they are being provided with. Their participation throughout any treatment or procedure is paramount, to attain an outstanding and positive outcome. Children and adolescents of military personnel may become foster children also. This happens when a service member is called to active duty. The children must, then be cared for by someone, other than the parent/care giver. This poses a unique situation because another degree of uncertainty arises. The children hope that their parents return back from what may be the theater of war. Thereby, experiencing diverse levels of emotional crisis. Every member of military service including but not limited by civilian childcare services will provide supportive psychological interventions.

The professionally licensed nurse, performing with empathy and an assertive approach, may facilitate the infant/child and nurse communication. However, to exude a sense of security, comfort and the understanding that the infant child responds to being accepted. Also, that their primary needs will be met, the infant child will, by nature, read or sense anyone in their presence. It is not only the infant but children from toddlers through young adulthood may use their instincts to deal with any traumatic situation. They may be traumatized when their normal milestones are interrupted.

It should be understood, that trauma, illness, disease and tragedy have no schedule and may occur at any time without notice. Therefore, the notice is, be as prepared as humanly possible. Take charge, when the moment arises "carpe diem". Perform within the scope of practice, being mindful of the boundaries and limitations, having a respect for all members involved and persons affected with professionalism, dignity, and respect.

You are assigned to collect specific blood and body fluids for drug and alcohol testing. The assignment requires boarding oil tankers and cargo ships. There are no other medical or nursing professionals on board. This is a unique situation. Now, the professionally licensed nurse, acting as an agent, for specific maritime and government office, is empowered to represent such entities. As an agent assigned to perform the collection of specimens for drug, alcohol and illicit substances, the professionally licensed nurse has become in charge of performing such service.

There will be other government representative present. These representatives are The United States Customs and Border Patrol agents, The United States Immigration, Customs Enforcement agents, Drug Enforcement Agency agent, The United States Coast Guard officer, the shipping and vessel agent. The appointed official agents are required by law to ensure that the proper legal methods of specimen collection are implemented. All of the ships personnel are to provide whatever specimen may be required for testing. Including all of the officers and operators of such assigned shipping vessels. If even one merchant marine became non-compliant, he would be repatriated for non-compliance and insubordination.

To board any shipping vessel, special government clearance is absolutely necessary. The ships may be anchored off shore. Which means that in order for the professional licensed practical nurse, as the representing drug and alcohol specimen collections agent, will need to be brought to the ship by, what is known as, a launch. The launch is a special water craft, like a water taxi, that the professional licensed practical nurse boards, after being cleared to board, and is then transported to the Oil tanker or cargo ship, at the location of anchorage. As smooth sailing as it appears, the ocean was not as calm as it seemed. Boarding ships with test collection equipment was not smooth either. Upon arriving to the ship to be boarded, depending on certain factor, the water currents and the location of the ship, a steady launch position had to be maintained.

There were times that the boarding of the ship was on the port side, the starboard side or from the bow or aft. If the ocean water was calm, a metal gangway would be lowered, for boarding the ship. The metal gangway was like a stairway with metal or rope handrails. If an oil tanker was full with oil for the oil tank transfer depot, it would be easy to board on to the deck of the oil tanker or cargo ships. That was because a fully loaded oil tanker would be lower to the water and the placement of the gangway would be on or closer to the launch. If the oil tanker or cargo ships were empty, the deck of the ship would be higher. In the case where the deck was not reachable by the gangway, or the oceans water was choppy and unsteady, the launch boat would be unsteady in the water. The launch boat would the bob up and down along side the ship. No matter what the water was like, the procedures for collection of specimens would have to be completed. Or else, the crewmembers would not be allowed to disembark, and would not be allowed to be on American soil. Therefore, a Jacobs' ladder would then be lowered off the side of a ship. The Jacobs ladder is a rope with wooden rungs secured onto the railings of the ship. Despite the strong and choppy current and the launch boat, alongside the ship, both bobbing on the ocean, with a medical pack on my back, I would have to climb up and onto the ships deck.

There would be maritime staff above on the ships deck, alongside the rails where the Jacobs ladder was secured. As I disembarked off of the launch boat and while climbing on the Jacobs ladder, to board onto the ships deck, the launch boat would be pressed up against the side of the ship, just below me, while climbed the Jacobs ladder, until I safely reached the ships deck and assisted onto the ships deck by the ships maritime staff. If there were no other ships to go to by the launch boat, the launch boat would wait until the collection of specimens were completed. It would take approximately an hour or two for the collection of specimens to be completed. Each crewmember would have to present their passports and appropriate merchant marine identification, which would be verified by the manifest and government agencies present on every ship. If the launch boat had to go to another ship, which may have been nearby, I would have to wait until the launch boat returned.

There were ships where the captain and officer would treat me exceptionally well. Since the officers mess hall, that is, the dining area on the ship, gets special treatment, with seven course meals served, and a gourmet chef, the officers would invite me to eat with them, while I waited for the launch boat to bring me back to shore. And they ate well. All of the ships were of international origin. There were times, aboard some ships that were manned by merchant marines of different countries. They did not speak English so a translator had to be assigned to me. The translators verified each crewmember with accurate presentation, for the thorough and accurate documentation and completion for the collection of specimens, to be tested for drug, alcohol and illicit substances. Some ships would be boarded at the oil refinery depots and secure docks.

When all of the specimens were collected and the accuracy of all required documents were verified, I would then have to disembark each ship. I would contact the launch boat dispatcher to confirm that all procedures were completed and verified, at which point I would board the launch boat. If a gangway could not be used for disembarking off the ship, I would then descend down the Jacobs ladder again. The completed collection of specimens from the ships crewmembers would then be prepared for shipment to the Department of justice drug testing centers or, in some situations, to the international police agencies from where the ships originated.

Anywhere on earth can become the workplace from where the professional licensed practical nurse would have to be assertive, take charge and get the work done. It could be on land, at a hospital, medical clinic, shopping center, library, house of worship, mobile vehicle, an airplane, jet or a ship on the ocean.

CHAPTER EIGHT

INDEPENDENT PRACTICE

On Your Own

INDEPENDENCE AND FREEDOM from institutional professional licensed practical nursing is only an application, a telephone call or an email away. Online pursuit of independent professional licensed practical nursing is also a matter of how prepared and confident the professionally licensed nurse is. When the licensed nurse is scheduled to be at a hospital or nursing home, there is a professional obligation and responsibility to be at such workplaces. Thereby, being a professional participant in providing professional medical and nursing care. Upon arriving at the clinical nursing unit, all providers of nursing care must gather together at the nurse's station for the endorsement of the nursing report, before and after every nursing tour. Since the nurses stations may be at an open area on the nursing unit, which is a HIPPA violation, a conference room or nurses lounge may suffice to hear the change of shift medical and nursing report. Even when making medical and nursing care patient rounds, by standing at the door of the patient/client room or at the patient/client bedside a HIPPA or PHI violation may occur.

Imagine what the patient/client may be thinking or imagining, by hearing the use of medical and nursing terminology. By such specialized medical communications, the patient/client may become scared and afraid of the unknown, which may produce psychological trauma. Although psychological trauma may have commenced upon the onset of illness or physical trauma, hearing such a different type of professional communication may be traumatizing. To prevent the traumatizing affect of the patient/client, a private and secure area for the endorsement of medical and nursing reports is paramount. Thereby, not producing psychological insult to the patient/client. This has been a reiteration and re-enforcement of protected health information (PHI) and HIPPA.

From birth and up until one becomes independent, we all yearn to be on our own, studying and practicing professionally on our own terms. The cliché "We must crawl before we walk" would be apropos, or by being taken by the hand through the journey of professionalism. The first requisite for independent professional nursing practice is a thorough knowledge of the tenets of nursing and clinical experience. There are several variations. How the licensed nurse acquires the professional license to practice nursing and develop professional experiences will determine how well the licensed practical nurse presents being confident of professional licensed nursing may depend on how well traveled and how well versed on practical nursing skills are expressed as well. Can you perform?

The first vehicle for the professional practice of licensed nursing is an established foundation of professional medical and nursing communication. Clear and concrete, verbal and written practice is paramount for independent professional licensed nursing practice, such as, body language, facial expressions, poise, diction and annunciation. No matter what your socio-cultural exposure has been, practice in professional medical and nursing performance can make or break your ability to be an independent practitioner of professional nursing.

With the licensure laws changing, there is a need for flexible and diverse professional licensed practical nurses. Caring for someone or a group is the professional desire of every nurse. Nursing is the most diverse profession of caring for all mankind. Therefore, establishing a solid foundation for independent professional nursing practice will require passion and dedication. There is primary clinical practice, specialty clinical practice, and community school practice, to mention a few. Every area of professional medical and nursing practice has its language. This may be synonymous to, from primary fuel to ultra fuel. The analogy of ultra fuel is when varied combinations and applications of professional medical and nursing communication are expressed.

The professionally licensed nurse may learn the primary and ultra methods of applied professional medical and nursing jargon. Although such applications are practice specific. Not all health care delivery personnel speak the same language. This is why areas of practice require specific qualifications in order to be able to deliver the proper standard of care. See "Standards of Care" in your country, state, city, locale, community and facility. Populations within a state, county or city will determine the standards of care. This is not to express a low or high standard of care, but to be prepared and able to apply licensed practical nursing theory with nursing practice. Furthermore, the standard of care will apply to the material tools, mechanical and pharmacological needs purchased for the professional delivery of medical and nursing practice. Applicable medical and surgical devices are provided with treatment and procedure standards for professional medical and nursing applications. Professional medical and surgical items and devices are made by different manufacturers, in the United States of America, and abroad. Be sure that you understand the indications, applications and the expected results of your tools.

As mentioned, your first tool is your ability to apply your licensed practical nursing knowledge professionally, comprehend primary and critical communications. The primary communication is that of the professional environment. Independent nurse practitioners (NP) will need special nursing credentials such as Pediatric Nurse Practitioner (PNP), Family Nurse Practitioner, (FNP) and nurse Midwife (NMW). In the military the licensed practical nurse will be classified by rank. Every aspect of the United States Armed Forces and its branches, that is, Army, Navy, Marines, Air Force and Coast Guard have their own identifying ranks and levels for the classification of military medical and nursing practitioners. From the medic, hospitalman, corpsman to medical specialists. At times performing independent of each other by the ranking Military Medical Director.

How, where and when does the professional licensed practical nurse perform and implement professional medical and nursing treatments and procedures independently? There is a fine-line that defines such independent practice by the professional licensed practical nurse. A private or public agency for the provision of professional medical and nursing practice may negotiate a contract, on behalf of the professional licensed practical nurse. Depending on the degree of advanced practical nursing education, training, certifications and licensure will determine how, if, when and where such independent practice by the professionally licensed nurse may be performed.

Reflecting on this example, upon attaining a professional licensed practical/vocational-nurse compact license, the licensed practical/vocational-nurse may travel and practice professionally at such state that recognizes and endorses the professional licensed practical/vocational-nurse for the professional practice of licensed nursing. Although, there may have to be a professionally licensed medical doctors' prescription or referral for the patient/client to be accompanied by a specially trained professionally licensed nurse. Depending on the actual professional medical and nursing needs for a specific patient/client may determine such prescribed need for professional nursing services. For this reason, the compact license was produced for such interstate licensed nursing practice. Thereby, also, opening the borders, boundaries and limitations for professional licensed practical/vocational nurses. This by no means implies that the professionally licensed nurse is totally autonomous. It simply states that as an integral member of the professional nursing process, the professionally licensed nurse performs under the supervision of the professionally licensed medical and nursing healthcare providers.

There are healthcare institutions, healthcare clinics and facilities in various states that recognize the professional licensed practical/ vocational-nursing license for professional practice at such healthcare institution, healthcare clinics and facilities public and private. Certain providers of professional medical and nursing agencies, organizations, corporations, companies, and government entities, public and private in such states, where the compact professional licensed practical/vocational-nursing practice are recognized. By attaining a professional affiliation with such agencies, organizations, corporations, companies and government entities, public and private is where particular standards of care are provided for the professional practice of licensed practical/vocational nursing. Therefore, as legally applicable, such agencies, organization corporations, companies and government entities, public and private, by the implementation of specific policies and procedures, established at participating states, where the performance of professional license practical/vocational- nursing is recognized.

Participating states which, recognize and endorse the professional licensed practical/vocational-nurse license, govern and regulate the compact license of the professional licensed practical/ vocational-nurse. The governance, rules regulations along with professional affiliations, establishes the independent professional nursing practices. As professionally customary, the professional licensed practical/vocational-nurse practice under the immediate supervision and management by the licensed medical doctor and/ or professional registered nurse. Though not so simply stated, let's take, for example, the mix of professional medical and nursing practice.

In 1989, a calamity occurred on the waters of the United States. Such calamity affected, not just the health and safety of the constituents of a state, but all of the wildlife in and on the waters and waterways and on land of the state. The affects of such a tragedy caused a tsunami throughout the world. An oil tanker, The Valdese, contracted by the Exxon oil company, hit an iceberg, off of the Prince William Sound of Alaska. The impact caused a massive gap to the ships oil tankers' oil tank that was filled with crude oil, which caused the ship to spill so much oil into the waters off of Alaska. Thereby, affecting an innumerable amount of wildlife in and on the water and waterways of Alaska. Affected also, was the wildlife on land including all of the citizens of the State of Alaska.

The massive ripple affect reached every country that ships any and all types of shipping vessels that ship any and all types of cargo, especially oil and oil based cargo. As a result, an integration of several government agencies, national, international, federal, state, local, public and private were created to monitor how products are shipped into American waters. The professional licensed practical nurse was also summoned to answer the call for the protection of all citizens, wildlife and waterways of The United States. Protections are mainly put in place to protect also all wildlife in and on the waters and waterways of The United States. Including the foul in the air, since, all nutrients for all humanity and wildlife are affected. That tragedy should never have happened. Therefore, unpredictable and unforeseen, whether by nature, human nature or the nature of things, may, for reasons unknown, produce the call for professionally licensed nurses to be answered. And the call was answered.

A corporation or company in New York State is affiliated with a government entity, such as the drug enforcement agency (DEA); the DEA is overseen by the international police agency (Interpol); a corporation, company or a private agency which provides licensed professional medical and nursing personnel at another state. For example, The State of California, by a negotiated contract, in New York State, and is affiliated with a private shipping company from a foreign country; the shipping company has specific cargo that has been cleared internationally by the governing entities of such foreign country, and is required to ship such cargo to New York State. The United States governing entity (DEA) is notified as well as the international governing entities (Interpol) of the shipping of such cargo that will be shipped to New York State from such foreign country but, needs to be internationally cleared to enter into the United States by way of international waters into The United States of America waterways for the shipping and delivery of such cargo. The agency which provides licensed professional medical and nursing personnel in New York State is contacted by the contracted agency in The State of California, which also provides licensed professional medical and nursing personnel, that a ship from a foreign country will be shipping cargo from a foreign country to the United States and will be shipped to New York State.

Before the cargo from the foreign country, which is on the ship from the foreign country, can be released at the shipping site in the State of New York, all maritime personnel must be legally cleared by specific government agencies and entities. A medical testing laboratory of specifically collected specimens at an independent location is notified by the governing entities of both the foreign country from where such ship and its cargo originate and the governing entities of the foreign ship and its cargo will be shipped to, to perform specific testing of such collected specimens at such notified independent medical testing laboratory; the independent medical testing laboratory then provides specific specimen collection equipment and documents for verification of such collected specimens which has been legally verified on the ship by the collecting agent which was deployed in New York State. The contracted agent in the State of New York is then notified by the contracting agency in the State of New York that specific medical testing equipment along within verifying documentation will be delivered to the contracting agency office location for pick up by the contracted agent who has been contracted in New York State.

Upon the picking up of such medical testing equipment and documents for verification of completed procedures of specific forensic specimen collection, the assigned agency contracted agent, who has conducted forensic specimen collection, is provided with all corporations, shipping company representative including representing government agents in New York State. At which time a date, time and location will be agreed upon, by all involved, for which the boarding of such ship for the collection, verification and completion of performance of procedures for collecting specific forensic specimens, are to be transported to a designated courier of such collected forensic specimens. The designated courier, that has also been legally cleared and charged with the possession and transport of such verified specific specimens to be tested at the laboratory where forensic testing of the specific specimens will be performed, will then ship the specimens to such designated forensic testing laboratory. Whereby, every agency, as well as, one involved, throughout the process of clearing the cargo ship and all personnel aboard the cargo ship, will perform such forensic verifications, by the signing of every document, from start to finish. The results the forensic testing of the specific specimens is confidential and will be filed with the owner of the country of origin of the shipping vessel. Inclusive, every government agency will also be informed.

As expressed, when becoming an independent professional licensed practical nurse, it essential to be prepared with the level and knowledge about what is to be performed, from appropriate education and training and to the related licensure and certifications thereof. There is a certain degree of professional responsibility, when performing independently, as a professional licensed practical nurse. There may not be a professionally licensed medical doctor or registered nurse in the immediate proximity at where the professional licensed practical nurse is perform medical or nursing treatments and procedures. Therefore, the professional licensed practical nurse, performing autonomously, will have, almost the full and complete responsibility for the outcomes of such treatments, procedures and professional communications.

As mentioned, independent, private and public agencies, which by dual representation, of professionally licensed and or certified medical and nursing professionals, negotiate specific contracts, for performing medical treatments at designated healthcare institutions, medical facilities and clinical settings. Because there are so many medical and nursing specialties, there are equally, if not more, specially educated and trained licensed nurses. It is virtually impossible to predict what kind of medical and nursing challenges may arise, even futuristically. Since tomorrow is promised to no one, how committed the professionally licensed nurse, to their nursing practice, it would be, more than just advisable and recommended that the professionally licensed nurse be diligent in keeping current and informed of what the licensed nurse is capable of accomplishing.

In contrast, the national and international legal rules and regulation for the testing of drug and substance abuse; a private corporation, with many variations and levels, of employees, may also be tested, by law, for drug, alcohol and substance abuse. By this anecdote, a large healthcare corporate agency, providing professional medical and nursing services will implement drug, alcohol and substance abuse testing of its employees. When a corporation employs such testing for drug, alcohol and substance abuse; the confidential and methodical implementation of having to test every employee and candidate for employment, poses a unique skill set by which to accomplish such a feat. In such incidence, coding, recoding and continual informal and regular indiscriminate rotation of testing and unannounced testing of every employee is paramount and essential. This occurred at one of the nationally large corporation of professional medical and nursing healthcare provisions.

Upon arrival, at a medical and nursing institution, facility, clinical setting, wherever it may be, it is expected the professionally licensed nurse be more than just freshly graduated from a school of practical nursing. It is expected, and not taken for granted, that upon accepting any assignment at any medical and nursing institution, health facility and clinical setting, that the licensed nurse is professionally prepared and ready to take charge of the assignments at such locations. It is expected, also, that the professionally licensed nurse be capable of acclimating and adapting to any and all conditions that may exist at any and all locations at which the professionally licensed nurse may be practicing as a professional nurse.

Truly, it is the complete and absolute obligation and responsibility of the licensed nurse to be, educated, trained and professionally prepared, especially for taking on professional medical and nursing contracted assignments. As is also, the complete and absolute obligation and responsibility of all involved in such contractual negotiations, where the performance of professional medical and nursing practices occur. The professionally licensed nurse is not totally and completely autonomous. When the professionally licensed nurse is assigned to perform remotely, that is, from home or in the field, for example; a professionally licensed medical doctor and or registered nurse may be assigned to directly supervise and oversee that the professional licensed practical nurse has been appropriately assigned specific professional medical and nursing assignments within the scope of professionally licensed nursing practice.

Because the professional licensed practical/vocational nurse is educated in medical and nursing terminology, professional medical communications are understood unilaterally, no matter from where in the world. Continually staying abreast of the professional medical and nursing documentation applications may also perform medical records reviews performed by the professional nurse. There are healthcare organizations and agencies, nationally, that provide general and specialty professional healthcare services. The provision of professional medical and nursing services are monitored and reviewed periodically. The review of professional medical and nursing patient/client records may also be reviewed for medical/legal applications. Therefore, any provider of professionally licensed medical or nursing treatments and procedures are obligated and responsible for the accurate and complete documentation of every type of communications, treatments and procedures that may have been administered and performed for every patient/client. Professional medical and nursing documentation may also include communications and referrals provided to the patient/client. Every professional medical and surgical specialty may have specific medical terminology relative to the type of medical and surgical specialty practice.

Throughout the country and the world, medical records require being reviewed. How, then, can the professional medical and nursing community measure and evaluate the performance of professional medical and nursing practices from outside of The United States? For these reasons, by the agreements of four internationally qualified medical entities were the international codes of diseases and disorders (ICD9/10) developed. Going forward, the ICD and medical compendium are continually updated, because of the discoveries in healthcare and the addition of cyber medical practices. By such professional medical and nursing practices, quantitatively and qualitatively, patient/client healthcare service may be provided, optimally. (See National, International Medical Record Review Public Health Laws Rules and Regulation in your state). Allied health providers may also be assigned to copy, extract and provide medical coding services, for the proper reviewing of medical records.

Medical records reviewed are governed by national, international, state and local government organizations. Because of the influx and migration of people from all over the world, specific national and international heath organizations, for example, the World Health Organization (WHO) in accordance with every nationality coming into the United States, have developed standards for the medical coding of illness, diseases and traumas that may affect individuals, communities and populations. (See World Health Organization). As a result of such human developments and interactions, the performance of professional medical records reviews may be conducted by the professional licensed practical nurse. The review of medical records and medical documents may be of the paper type of medical documents, computerized type of medical documentation or of a combination of both paper and electronic medical records (EMR).

The professional licensed practical nurse may perform medical record reviews remotely from the comfort of their home, which is pretty cool, at a hospital, medical clinic or at a doctors' office. There may be a team of nurses to preform medical records reviews together, where the professionally licensed nurse participates at such medical records reviews. Medical coding and abstraction may be included in the performance of the reviewing of medical records. Whether from the comfort of home, at a medical institution, medical clinic or doctors' office, strict adherence to HIPPA and PHI laws, rules and regulates must be observed. It is not unusual that the professional review of medical records may include reviewing medical record from foreign countries. When presented with medical records of foreign countries, there must be supporting interpreted medical documentation accompanying such foreign medical documents, for the proper, accurate and professional medical records review to be verified as a professional and appropriate medical records review.

The review of medical records will require specific education and training of medical coding and use of the international codes of diseases (ICD 10). To understand and interpret ICD codes and modifiers that are documented in the medical records it is essential that the professional licensed practical nurse also become an expert with the applications of the ICD 10. There is also another medical coding application. That is, the application of clinical procedures and treatment codes (CPT) codes. ICD and CPT codes are unique and different and not interchangeable or inter-applicable of each other for applications by professional medical and healthcare providers. Depending on the styles of professional medical, surgical and therapeutic practitioners may determine the applications of such medical and therapeutic codes.

There are various types of medical records reviews that may be performed independently by the professional licensed practical nurse with the coordination and over read review by the professional registered nurse. Depending on the level and type of medical review, whether quarterly, seasonal or annually. The contracted organization will provide the professionally licensed nurse with all necessary computer equipment and procedure manuals for the performance of such medical records reviews. Whereby, the professional and accurate review of medical records may be reviewed, accordingly.

Whether contracted to assist with professional clinical medical and nursing procedures in the occupational health services department or the organ transplant department; within a hospital, a specially integrated level of professional healthcare education and training is paramount. The occupational health services department has its own and unique set of clinical applications of treatments and procedures. Employee health services are not provided for employees only but also for potential employees. Employee health surveillance and monitoring services are implemented by the regularly monitoring and scheduling of its' employees. After all, the maintenance of employee health status is paramount for optimal profession performance by every employee. Including the professionally contracted at the medical institution where they work at.

Military personnel are not the exception, as being an employee, so to speak. Because of the military service to The United States of America, the term of "Servicemen" would be appropriately applied. Therefore, the surveillance and monitoring of the health and welfare each and every military serviceman would be an absolute responsibility by the United States of America, here at home and abroad. That being expressed, where an eminent heath danger may exist, it is the responsibility of the employer to provide professional health services for its employees. Whereby, such health monitoring, not only the place at which an employee is employed may be negatively affected or impacted, but also the community at where the employee lives and commutes through.

In 1980, an unknown and unidentified disease presented itself among the human race. While being employed at a private hospital in New York City, the impact on every employee, professional and ancillary, was intense. It was a time that when a person became affected by such an unknown disease, the affected person and persons life was cut so short it frightened, not just the employees of that hospital, but the entire world. Including the military and all nations. Affected persons, then, may have lived for up to two or three days, since no medical treatments were available. Because of such impact on the world, the professional healthcare community implemented the health monitoring of every employee and potential employee, including healthcare contractors.

Rigorous professional health education and training was provided for every employee, patient/client and contractors. By having every one of the professional and non-professional providers of healthcare aware of such an epidemic, several campaigns arose against the proliferation of the biological viral affects on the whole world. When such a viral impact on the world was identified, a strong and impactful approach against such proliferation of a dangerous virus was launched. From music artists, television and stage performers, the message, by way of any and all forms of media was delivered. From Europe to The United States and to the entire human race, and not limited to farmers, entomologists and the veterinary community, everyone was made aware of such a devastating disease. Anyone or anything could be a vector of such disease. The Center for Disease Control (CDC) and the World Health Organization (WHO) played a major and impactful role on the world.

Employees and servicemen alike were regularly tested and monitored as a result of such a proliferation of such a viral disease. Commonly equated with the plague or typhoid, where a pandemic becomes an epidemic. Initially identified as a viral disease and after vigorous and rigorous scientific research of such a biological danger to humanity, the Human Immune Virus (HIV) was identified and the after affects, combined with other diseases and disorders, such as, Acquired Immune Disease Syndrome (AIDS) effective medical treatments and procedures have been implemented. The brave and bold professional medical and nursing community played a strong and important role in the support of controlling and preventing an epidemic of biblical proportion.

I paid close, like fly paper close, attention to the affects of such a viral disease that, to this date, became a life long and impactful lesson for me. First and foremost, I thank The Lord, for providing me the opportunity for providing professional licensed practical nursing care to the first and many of children, adults, their families and significant loved ones affected by such an indiscriminate biological virus. The Professional medical, nursing, scientific as well as every ancillary personnel, at that time, played an astute and responsible role throughout the healthcare process. Special and specific treatments, procedures and protocols were developed and strictly implemented. Every precaution, with no stone unturned, was implemented, thereby, providing protections for the affected patient/client, staff, employees and the communities of such employees and their families.

The ripple affects and to date, created by such a disease, have opened new and greater possibilities for the practice of professional licensed practical nursing. This is not to imply that it takes a problem to cement the practice of licensed practical nursing amongst the professional medical and nursing community, but to support the professional and nursing community as well as any and all professional providers of healthcare. From an educational standpoint and not limited to communities and the world.

It has been approximately four decades that such a biological attack on humanity and the world has been realized and just over three decades that effective medical treatments have been implemented. It is hoped that a cure be realized as well as an improvement of the quality of life for all. Until then, it is imperative and of the utmost importance that humanity and the entire professional medical, nursing, scientific and non-medical and scientific communities forge on for such a cure. Inclusively, the professional licensed practical nurse will be an important and integral member of the professional medical and nursing community for the implementation and professional performance of medical treatments and procedures, professionally prescribed, for each and every person without prejudice or reservation.

CHAPTER NINE

NURSE CONTRACTOR/VENDER

BUSINESS AND POLITICS have the same void as the oceans. Although the oceans are connected fluidly, sea life and the waters support earth and the people's lives that depend on the nature what the waters provide for the sustenance of humanity. If you cannot swim you drown. The currents of the waters are always changing direction. Through the changing currents are also the changing tides. There is no true measurable pulse of the oceans, rivers or lakes. Not even of the puddles left behind. There is no heart in the waters that an electrowatergraph can be applied to. Not even by satellite. Although there is a rhythm and a flow of all waterways, there are no aquatic emotions of any waterway. If the waters had emotions, people and water vessels would never sink. As a U.S. Navy Veteran, I have learned to respect the waterways, especially, the body and rhythms of the oceans. Like being cradled by tender waterways. Therefore, if the waters are not understood, no one should be having any business on or in them.

In contrast to the waterways, business have no measurable vital signs, short of Wall Street. So we look at the balance of the waters and the balance of business. Which brings to mind the law of supply and demand. People are living longer and by the nature of things produce the demand for professional quality and outstanding healthcare. But since business is emotionless, the professional challenge, by the licensed nurse, is up to provide and fill the emotionless gap with the professionalism of empathy and genuine TLC. The demand for professionally licensed nurses can be met. To produce the supply that would meet the demand of professionally licensed nurses, will require the support of every state in the nation.

When it comes to politics, it is best to research how politics applies to the professional licensed practical nurse. Since Juris Prudence has no emotions as well. It would seem that to be emotionless is to be heartless. It really does take heart. It takes a lot of heart to provide care for anyone suffering from a traumatic experience. By that reality, this is a treasure of empathy, which lives in the hearts of all professional medical and nursing providers of healthcare. To provide such an outstanding quality of service to humanity, the licensed nurse, without political influence, is professionally prepared and geared up for incredible outcomes.

The professional nurse may be contracted, by any organization that is in need of healthcare, which may be performed by the professionally licensed nurse. Providing, that there is a licensed medical doctor acting as the medical director, on the board of directors, in support of healthcare practices for the corporation, company or any organization, by design. This is not limited to a single person in need or a corporation or business entity providing health services. So long as the licensed practical nurse practices within the guidelines of the nurse practice act. There does not need to be a licensed registered nurse present. When licensed nurses practice professionally at all nursing levels, the practice of nursing professionally, will be always by the direction of, a licensed medical doctor, which legally, will be required. In the team approach, there will also be a professionally licensed registered nurse. All nurses are required to be, whether by direct or indirect, supervised by a licensed medical doctor.

Providing health services to anyone, by definition, is a service that can be provided to anyone as a vendor, thereby, delivering healthcare services to the healthcare recipient. As stated in Chapter one, the healthcare recipient may be a private person a nursing agency or registry, a corporation or facility, that is, an institution, a school or a community. Financial rates and fees will vary from recipient to recipient as well as the degree of health service provided. (See private independent practice rules and regulations in your state).

The professionally licensed nurse contractor/vendor is a duly licensed nurse in the state of practice of where the license to practice nursing at the practical nurse level, has been attained. Supported by a licensed medical doctor and the professional medical and nursing team. The licensed practical/vocational nurse can be contracted to meet the demand of healthcare services. Professionally licensed nurse contracts may be represented and negotiated by an agency that represents professionally licensed medical and nursing healthcare providers.

Networking with persons in need of nursing care, corporations or communities is necessary for success as an independent licensed practical nurse contractor. A licensed nurse can start their private business. Advertising by word of mouth, are the best modes for successfully becoming a professionally licensed nurse contractor. First the licensed nurse would need to have documented experience, appropriate credentials, a good list of evaluations and references. Who knows, your practice might even enter the Fortune 500 level. Wishful thinking.

The term vendor is defined as a person, group, corporation, manufacturer, company or a community that provides goods and/or services or products to a person, group, corporation, manufacturer, company or community, requesting such goods and or services in exchange for a fee. Goods or products may be tangible such as band aides, or any manufactured item or manufactured device. Inclusive of such products are, in the case of licensed nursing, the standard and or specialized professional licensed practical nursing knowledge and acquired experience by the professional performance and implementation of such standard an or specialized professional nursing practices. The provision of professional services, goods or products in possession by the licensed nurse is by the performance, implementation, and evaluation, quantitatively, of such standard or specialty professional licensed nurse education, training and or acquired experience.

Who would think that the attainment of an education would become a product? In contracts, there are paragraphs with divisions of paragraphs, and sub division of paragraphs in which exists the definition of products and services, with levels and degrees of such defined products and services. Inclusive are the chapters in which such paragraphs reside and may also be defined, as are the paragraphs, where products and services may be introduced. (In chapter ten I will go somewhat further as to how and when this paragraph applies.) Therefore, in the same way the professionally licensed nurse studied and prepared to become a licensed nurse, whereby, diligently applying oneself for becoming a professionally licensed nurse; with the same and more variably and diverse stringent diligence, in the acquisition of brilliant professional nurse product. As a cliché may imply, "a person may become a product of their environment". With a little tenacity, the professional licensed practical nurse may become an outstanding vendor of their acquired product and services.

Usually, an independent agency and its agents, who provide the products and services of licensed professional medical and nursing practitioners, may solicit such professional medical and nursing services to corporations, groups, companies, institutions, medical clinics and government entities. The private or public agency may also solicit an accompanying contract, by which to negotiate the products and services, which pertain to, the requested products and services by corporations, groups, companies, institutions, medical clinics and government entities.

On January of 1990, by the Presidential Order of President George W. Bush, of the United States Navy, I was mobilized for active duty military Service. It was an activation of my specialized military medical education and training to be implemented for Operation Desert Storm/Desert Shield. At which time, all of my specialized medical military education and training kicked in. I was advanced to the rank of Leading Petty Officer of Military Medicine, an extraordinary level of medical healthcare practice. I was mobilized to a submarine base where I was specially educated and trained to orient, educate and train specific levels, rates and ranks of military medical personnel. There is a rigid chain of communication by which every military medical process is performed. All branches of military personnel, including affiliated civilian personnel and their families were to be provided healthcare services at varying degrees. It was an arduous and intense implementation of theory by which to perform military medical services. Therefore, specialized educated and trained military medical and administrative personnel were mobilized.

In order to provide outstanding and exemplary healthcare service, the specialized educated and trained corpsman, hospitalman and administrative medical personnelman, followed specific military medical orders, that is, every military medical order, which was prescribed by the Captain of Military Medicine, Military Medical Corps. Such military medical orders were to be delegated through the ranks of specific military personnel. From the ranks of military personnelman and through the ranks military medical corpsman, the implementation of every prescribed order, given to every rank of military personnel, was carried out precisely and effectively. Professionally known as The Chain of Command. Reversely, the supervision and evaluation of every prescribed military medical order, implemented and performed was meticulously reviewed before, during and after each prescribed military medical order. Included in the reviewing of military medical healthcare service, which were provided to military servicemen, their families and civilian personnel are unique rates and ranks of all branches of The United States Armed Forces, reviewing and storing such military medical records and documents. Military servicemen are always transitioning, nationally and internationally. Therefore, accurate documentation and storage of military medical records must accompany all servicemen to wherever their designated destination may be, including the theater of war and crisis.

By implementing such methods, procedures and processes through the civilian channels of professional healthcare, outstanding, exemplary and positive outcomes may be achieved. Although, in the course of providing military healthcare services, there are, also, the civilian public and private contractor which may also be integrated in to providing goods and services for The United States Armed Forces. It would seem a tangle, by such intricate military and civilian affiliations. It is by the clear and concrete negotiations of specific contracts for goods and services, where this type of marriage of government and civilian relationship may be achieved. There is a plethora of healthcare contracts, throughout the world. It is not expected, that all professional providers of healthcare products and services, be completely well versed of such contracts. Because of such of a plethora of legal contracts, there are specifically and professional educated and trained agents that negotiate such professional and specific contracts for the provision of professional medical and nursing goods and services.

Before choosing to go solo, it is absolutely advisable and necessary to explore, try, and become familiar with the multitude and variations of professional healthcare delivery systems. There are multitudes of professional healthcare delivery systems to choose from. Besides, clinical nursing practice may be treated as goods and services provided, performed and implemented by the professionally licensed nurse. There are also businesses that provide durable medical equipment. Besides providing durable medical, some equipment is expendable, that is, periodically and or frequently disposed, repaired, refurbished and reordered. Throughout the professional medical and nursing process, home infusion therapy monitoring may be provided to the patient/client. Which translates into that, not only is the patient/client receiving infusion therapeutic monitoring, but also the infusion devices are also monitored. All throughout the professional medical and nursing process. Thereby, placing the total responsibility of patient/client and therapeutic devices monitoring on the independent professional licensed practical nurse in charge.

Every professional medical institution, be it a hospital, nursing home, rehabilitation facility, medical clinics including and not limited to doctor's offices may be responsible for the ordering and the implementation of therapeutic medical equipment and medical devices. The medical doctor may also order therapeutic medication and nutritional fluids. Specific fluids, such as, intravascular medications, may be for therapeutic infusion, with the application of an electronic medication infusion device. There are also, parenteral nutritional therapeutic devices. All therapeutic medical devices and therapeutic fluid medications and nutritional fluids will require monitoring by a specially educated and trained licensed medical and or nursing professional. This may include the ordering and implementation of professional licensed practical nurses who are professionally educated and trained; for monitoring therapeutic medications and enteral nutritional infusion by such therapeutic infusion devices. Inclusively, there may be respirators, bariatric and many other specialized medical and surgical therapeutic devices.

Therefore, the professionally licensed nurse may become a representative of the manufacturer or supplier of durable medical equipment and products. Not just a representative of such durable medical equipment and devices, but also a trainer of such durable medical equipment and products. By this anecdote, when the specialized monitoring of the diabetic patient/client, with the implementation of specialized electronic devices became necessary: at hospitals, medical clinic and nursing home, one of the first companies which manufactured and produced such diabetic blood testing and monitoring devices, specially educated and trained professionally licensed nurses were contracted. Instructing and training professional medical and nursing personnel, at every level, were educated and trained in the use and implementation of glucometers, glucose reagent for the accuracy of glucometers, blood glucose testing strips and accurate documentation and monitoring of diabetic blood glucose. This specialized diabetic blood glucose testing and monitoring education and training was performed in New York City, New York by a contracted licensed practical nurse. The specialized education and training of the blood glucose testing, monitoring and accurate documentation was implemented at hospital nursing in-service and education sessions on several specialty clinical areas within each hospital. The general medical and nursing units, emergency room departments, labor and delivery units, intensive care, stepdown intensive care, coronary care, stepdown coronary care and telemetry units, pediatric units as well as at doctor's offices and point of care medical clinics. Diabetic devices education and training was implemented at Veterans Administration hospital and clinics, state and community hospital and clinics. Inclusive of such specialized prescribed in depth education and training were the laboratory technicians and pathologists on the accession of the national and international documentations, evaluation communications monitoring of diabetic patient/clients.

Before any medical and nursing equipment, device, medication or medically invasive product or therapeutic medication is prescribed by a licensed medical doctor, surgeon or nurse practitioner; the Food and Drug Administration (FDA) and or the United States Pharmacopeia Administration (USPA) must approve such medical and surgical therapeutic medical equipment, devices, medications and enteral nutritional fluids. Wherefore, such approval by the FDA the USPA by an underwriters laboratory approval (UA) testing conditions and laboratory usage, for human prescription, implementation and consumption. The protection and safety of everyone in proximity and implementation is paramount. For example, also, upon pursuing professional enhancements for becoming flexible and diverse, as well as, multi-marketable, the professionally licensed nurse, will be educated and trained, in depth, on the use and implementation of the electrocardiograph, blood and body fluid evacuation tube set (ETS) for professional safety and implementation. Inclusive, may also be the specialized education and training of the insertion of intravenous infusion catheter device (ICD) set for intravenous fluid infusion therapy and or the extraction of venous blood.

Sometimes it would take an exceptionally, educationally and experientially trained licensed professional nurse, to perform and implement a unique set of diversified, education, training and experience, although, to acquire such diverse education, training and experience can take some time. To develop such professional licensed practical nursing experience would actually take not one or two years. It would take anywhere from ten, twenty and even thirty or more years of professional medical and licensed practical nursing at varying areas and levels, inclusive, of highly, intensive specialized education and training of the professionally licensed nurse. Included in having such experience is a solid sense of professional discipline, mature demeanor, integrity and respect of self and others. There are professional medical and nursing professionals who can surf and professional medical and nursing professional that can surf. And there are those who just skate.

Sink or swim, the dedicated and prepared licensed practical nurse can make it to shore. The term "to shore", analogous for meaning, "to hold up the fallen, the broken, the weak and infirm"; like when a wall and a beam appears weak or weakening, shoring up the weak and weakening wall or beam can make all the difference between tragedy, casualty and calamity. Therefore, because a chain is only as strong as its weakest link, so is a licensed medical and nursing professional as capable as its fellow colleague. The lifeline and primary instrument of every professional, no matter what may be the profession, is the professional jargon/language and its application thereof. The environment is as important as, for where applicable, the positive, outstanding, exemplary and quality outcomes, quantitatively, and qualitatively that will tell the story clearly and transparently. In the medical and nursing chain of events, every medical, nursing student and healthcare professionals are just as an integral member of the medical and nursing teams and its coordinating counterparts.

CHAPTER TEN

MEDICAL-LEGAL ASPECTS

Let's Be Clear

"To paraphrase a quote by President Abraham Lincoln."
"A Nurses Talent, Time and Advise is Their Stock in Trade"

L AWS, STATUTES, CODES, rules and regulations are what make up the roads traveled that all businesses, professions, professionals, for everyone, in society as a whole. With so many layers of law, statutes, codes, rules and regulations, the professionally licensed nurse must be aware of the boundaries and limitations that govern the practice of the licensed nurse. Every applicable law will dictate how, when and where the professional licensed practical nurse may perform. Inclusive, are the civilian ramifications that, also, present unique boundaries and limitations which, may affect the civilian as well as the professional environment of healthcare professionals. This brings to mind, "The Good Samaritan Law".

Not everyone is familiar or knowledgeable of how the Good Samaritan Law applies to providers of healthcare. Briefly, "The Good Samaritan Law" is not a get out of trouble free law. The Good Samaritan Law may apply to people who are indigenous or not educated or knowledgeable of Public Health Laws (PHL). Particularly civilians, who are not educated or trained in life saving treatments and procedure; Therefore, anyone educated or trained in life saving treatments or procedures, such as in, cardio pulmonary resuscitation (CPR) may not be immune to a negligence or mal-practice violation. Including any instructors of healthcare education and training or where the provision of health services is performed.

It is virtually impossible to become omniscient of every law on earth. Respectively, there are schools where specific and applicable laws are taught. To be more specific, healthcare laws, statutes, codes, rules and regulation, with noted boundaries and limitation, are introduced to students of practical nursing. Narrowing the introduction of such laws, statutes, codes, rules and regulations to the professionally licensed nurse, may provide somewhat of an understanding of how, where and when such laws, statutes, codes, rules and regulations affect the professionally licensed nurse. Although, every licensed provider of healthcare may have such legal definitions, respective of the type and level of professional medical and nursing, an awareness of such definition of laws is essential.

As described, the laws of professional healthcare practices may seem vague and unclear. Courses of applicable medical and nursing laws are offered to every licensed professional medical and nursing practitioner. There are approximately three hundred plus type and levels of law. Within each type and level of law are divisions and sub-divisions of law. Therefore, because of what seems legally complicated, there are specific specialty lawyers in the practice specific and specialty medical, nursing, healthcare and public health law. It would seem confusing as to what legal specialist one would seek for legal advise or counsel. Narrowing such pursuit for such medical and nursing advise and counsel is a matter of what clearly may medically need to be addressed.

When I hit the legal wall, upon advice of my brother, who specialized in legal research, I enrolled in a paralegal course at The New York City Trial Lawyers Association, in downtown New York City, New York. There, I was introduced to the halls of law. What a ravel. Well not really. The instructors were all practicing Attorney's at Law. Although, there are fundamentals of law, the specifics from where legal fundamentals are drawn from will depend on who and how legal actions are presented. Therefore, let it be known, that every legal situation and case is unique. Although a legal case may seem alike or the same as an action brought on by anyone, in actuality, it is not.

From after having chosen an attorney for who a specific legal case is commenced until the case is closed, there are several steps involved. For the purposes of understanding legal cases of negligence or mal-practice, a brief narrative would be in order. First, lets explore some legal foundations. Comparatively, the professional language of medicine and nursing may be applicable to professional applications of law as specific legal jargon and terminology. Although the origin of legal language is specific to the level and type of law practiced, the actual origin of legal terminology is Latin and Greek. Something like medical terminology but more like critical thinking. Inclusive, the vehicle language of law is the language of the country, culture and or traditions. For this expository explanation, it would be English.

There is the compendium of Civil Practice Laws and Rules (CPLR, Domestic Relations Law (DLR), Real Property Law (RPL), Contract Laws and Rules (CLR), Criminal Procedures and Practice (CPP), to mention a few and Corporation Law Procedure (CLP) and Public Health Law (PHL). Within the, aforementioned, types and levels of law practiced are, also, the mechanisms of legal language and the applications thereof. As previously stated, every legal action has a beginning and an end. Or so it appears. Before the commencement of a legal action the identification and consent of the persons involved will be necessary.

Contracts and agreements seem similar in that someone or a company makes an offer. The offer may seem attractive. Therefore, the person or company that was made the offer to engage in the discussion of such offer. Both sides discuss plausible outcomes. But eventually, becomes a negotiation. Both sides would like to be the winner. Except only one would like to be the victor. Actually, a win win outcome would seem more favorable. Actually, there are two types of contracts. One being expressed on a written document, that is, where terms and conditions exist. The other is a verbal contract sealed by a handshake. Otherwise known as a parole contract. The former being legal and binding and the latter changing as time goes by. The only way a parole contract can be binding is if a witness was present at the time of such parole contract was introduced.

The legal and binding contract (The Agreement) is a more detailed agreement with specifics. Almost like a will or a stipulation of agreement as by and between both parties. Unless appropriately and legally represented and documented, always read every document where your signature or initials are embodied on. If you do not understand the legal language or vocabulary, ask for an explanation. Otherwise, entering blindly into any agreement may cost your license, your career as well as your future. At the point of adulthood, it is taken for granted, that everyone knows what he or she is doing. Thereby, taking on the responsibility of what might be an unknown and poorly negotiated agreement.

Patient/clients always seem grateful for healthcare services provided to them. In the moment of such elation, the patient/client feels that a gift would be a good way of showing their gratitude. Usually, there are no strings attached. Sealed with the handshake. Not so fast. As a professional licensed practical nurse, we do not walk around with contracts for everyone to sign. Therefore, it is essential to be clear when communicating with the patient/client. Upon entry to care, the client/patient may sign specific forms, which expresses their consent to have healthcare provided for them. The standard terms and conditions expressed. Also, that the patient/client may refuse at anytime when healthcare is being provided. Known as the Patient Bill of Rights.

I will repeat and reiterate, even if the patient/client is a friend or family member, no parole contract should ever be entered into. Probate and Surrogate law is a very sensitive area of law, which may require detailed descriptions of how the patient/client will be represented. By this interpretation, it is best to have a contract of

Proxy in the patient/client medical records. Never, by no means, accept any gift of real estate or real property from any patient/client. Not even if it is gifted by a family member or loved one. By accepting such gifts of apparent gratitude are where strings or even chains are born. No institution of healthcare includes such gifting in the agreement for healthcare contract. A humble thank you will always suffice for the gratitude expressed by the patient/client. A shared and victorious moment will go a long way. The true win win.

While practicing a renowned and prestigious hospital, a patient, who was being treated for a terminal illness, was being treated exceptionally well by all hospital staff members. The family of this patient/client was very pleased by how this patient/client was cared for. How the patient/clients spirit was lifted. Day after day, despite the client/patients state of health, the patient/client and the family took specific notice of a staff member. This staff member was not a nurse or therapist. The staff member was an environmental maintenance worker. Who, while cleaning the patient/client room, would talk sports and team outcomes with the patient/client. It was the evening shift, just after the six o'clock news. The patient/client state of mind was not always in tune with the six o'clock news, since the sports portion of the news was short, to a few minutes.

Day after day, the patient/client looked forward to engaging in conversational sports talk with the staff member, since it would take a little longer than a sports news moment. The patient/client seemed pleased and looked forward to engaging with the staff member. The family spoke awesomely well of having witnessed the interactions of all staff. Unfortunately, the day came to pass, when the client/patient expired, the family wanted to express their gratitude to the entire staff, specifically, the housekeeping person, for being exceptionally attentive. They wanted to give him a gift of gratitude. The nurses advised the family that it should be presented at the nurse's station. It was a very expensive watch.

To avoid the embarrassment of litigation, upon arrival to the patient unit, just before the six o'clock news, the housekeeping staff member was asked to be at the nurse's station. All of the unit staff, doctors, nurses and ancillary staff were present. The family, with the sincerest of emotion and gratitude, presented the gift of gratitude, in the presence of all staff members to the housekeeping member. It was an emotional moment of surprise, for all the staff, especially for the housekeeping staff member. We were all glad that this presentation, by the patient/client family, occurred on the unit, at the nurse's station.

This goes to show that one does not need to be a nurse to bring about comfort and caring to a patient/client. But as witnessed publically, no specific agreement was entered into by anyone. By surprise and spontaneity, an unexpected member of the healthcare team was recognized. The takeaway was that when least expected by anyone, the patient/client and family took notice of such integrated staff interaction and caring.

Besides, civil law practice, there are also, maritime, aerospace and military law practitioners. The practice of maritime law is an intricate type and levels of laws, which requires how to understand navigating national and international waters. Inclusively, the Atlantic Ocean, Pacific Ocean, Caribbean Sea, Mediterranean Sea, The China Sea, The Gulf of Mexico, The Persian Gulf, Great Lakes, Mississippi River, Hudson and East Rivers, Panama Canal and related waterways. Since our planet Earth is sixty six percent water, it would stand to reason that, an enumerable type and levels of maritime laws can be quite challenging. Simply expressed, when a water vessel is manufactured and commissioned, certain legal levels of operations of such vessel are implemented. The cruise liner ship will have professionally educated and trained staff on aquatic medical emergency treatments, procedures and protocols. The same applies to cargo ocean vessels, for example, with the exception of legal mandates. Due to the implementation of the Valdes Law, referencing an accident/incident, which occurred off the coast of Alaska, when by the negligence of the official maritime merchant marines, oil was spilled into the coastal waters of Alaska. That oil spill affected the Alaskan eco-systems, fowl, fish and wild life as well as the citizens of Alaska. The repercussions of such incident reverberated throughout the world. As a result of such an egregious event, the staff and officers for every commissioned water vessel is by law, mandated to be tested for drug, alcohol and substance abuse. I had the honor of being a representative agent for the government agencies, national and international as well as local entities, in the collection of specimens for drug, alcohol and substance abuse. For the sole purpose of keeping The United States of America and all affiliate shipping vessels safe from such negligent incidents. Having served in The United States Navy prepared me on what to expect when assigned being on ships with various types of cargo.

The plaintiff(s) is the person group or entity that brings a complaint against the person, group or entity being complained about. By such commencement, the plaintiff seems to have a complaint against who or what is identified as the defendant. When a defendant is brought into the legal arena, the burden of proof will be on the plaintiff. Because a legal action is commenced, does not mean there will always be a winner. Therefore, the merits of any commencement of any legal issue will go through, and with due diligence, a legal process. That legal process may be that the legal responsibility and obligations of the attorney, whom chosen and retained, by a litigant, the plaintiff. Because the burden of proof is on the plaintiff, it is of paramount clarity and importance, that the plaintiff must be absolutely clear and certain that their complaint have merit. Just because someone experiences an insult of sorts does not mean that they should commence legal action that may not be of or have merit.

Sometimes, going through the motions of legal consultation may provide such details where it would be improper to commence any legal action. In certain situations there may exist ambiguity or equivocation that may deem a legal action null and void of any merit and not legally viable. Upon a clear and certain belief that the commencement of a legal action has merit, certain legal documents are required. First and foremost, the plaintiff(s) signs an affidavit or retainer, which expresses and describes the terms and primary agreement by and between the plaintiff(s) and the attorney(s) for which the commencement of legal action where costs and disbursements are negotiated. Which is customarily thirty three percent plus legal costs and disbursements. Upon the discussion, and review of evidence and legal document, by the attorney or the their legal team, the following legal documents and affidavits may be obtained, from the plaintiff(s); Affidavit for the release of medical records, affidavits of legal service, specific affidavits for motion practice, such as continuance or certain points of release and or negotiated stipulation.

A summons and complaint is crafted on behalf of the plaintiff(s) to be served on the defendant. The Summons and complaint may be amended at some point after the initial service. Application for commencement of such legal action must be filed with the court or county clerk at where the legal action has been commenced. An identifying court index or docket number is purchased and assigned to the legal action, which appears on all legal documents pertaining to action filed in such court. A request for jury intervention (RJI) application may also be filed with the summons and complaint in the court where the legal action has been commenced, for the purpose of tracking the legal action through the legal processes. A variation of applicable subpoenas will be, as legal instruments, implemented for the acquisition of legal evidence. Before going forward on the merits of the legal action, a response or legal answer by the defendant must be received by the attorney for the plaintiff. Most times, the attorney for the defendant may stipulate denial of such complaint or statements of the complaint therein.

There will be inspection of legally obtained documents, such as medical records, employment records, financial records, premises and location record, photographs, film, video and recorded documentation for discovery of pertinent meritorious evidence in support of the plaintiff(s) legal action (D&I). Plaintiff and defendant medical, surgical and psychological examinations may be performed. The legally assigned board certified medical, surgical and psychiatric and psychological providers of performing such legally assigned medical, surgical physicals and psychiatric examinations will provide the plaintiff and defendant attorneys such medical, surgical, psychiatric and psychological finds. This type of diagnostic evaluative process will further be examined by the insurance medical professional for determining the merits and legal implications of such legal action, brought on by the attorney for the plaintiff(s). It is not unusual that several, board certified, medical, surgical, psychiatric and psychological healthcare providers are entered into such an extensive legal action.

After all, the plaintiff(s) attorneys will legally try and put up meritorious fight for the plaintiff(s), to produce a favorable judgment and favorable verdict and monetary award. Respectively, the defense attorney or defense team representing the defendant(s) may put up a meritorious defense, so as not to incur the responsibility of a legal judgment against the defendant(s). After all, everyone in any legal action wants to be the victor.

Medical, professional, corporate or vehicle Insurances, when applicable may also be implemented and filed at the court venue where the legal action has been commenced. A Bill of Particulars (BOP) is crafted by the attorney for the plaintiff(s), which indicate and describes the injuries, losses and effects on the plaintiff(s), as well as, legal requests to the court for judgment, verdict and relief on behalf of the plaintiff(s). Also, an attorney for the plaintiff(s) should have a proficient trial attorney on board. Just as what glitters may not always be diamonds, equally so, having a law degree may not always apply to every legal action. After all, a dentist cannot fix your car.

However long it takes to get through such litigation will depend on specific and particular statutes of limitations, which form the commencement of the legal action and responses throughout the legal actions of a case. If a case has immediate and verifiable evidence, the legal doctrine of, "res ispa loqutor", may be invoked, by the attorney for the plaintiff(s). Which, in Latin, by definition, states, "the thing speaks for itself ". Whereby, when invoked may hurry up the legal action. Equally, if the Latin legal term is invoked, that is, "res judicata", which by Latin legal definition, indicate that, based on the merits of the legal action, the assigned judge, may hurry up the judgment, verdict and relief on behalf of the plaintiff(s). Amongst other legal doctrine of law, which may also be invoked. Either way, it becomes a lengthy legal process. The courts require so many steps per legal process. To prove due diligence and without typo's, even a typo can make all the difference between the merits, legal review, process of service, court and attorney legal services agencies and the court clerk, for reaching a conclusion of a legal action. Hopefully, with diligent calendar practices, the attorney for the plaintiff(s) might just attain a speedy conclusion.

That was only a brief synopsis of what may be involved, upon the commencement of a legal action of a personal injury court case. Since every legal action of a personal injury matter is different and unique, consulting the right attorney(s) for legal action is essential to any case. At the attorneys' office, there may be a legal library for the aggregation of comparative legal cases in support of a legal action. Since every case is different and unique, the legal research involved will need to obtain strong and viable legal history documented for similar and comparative legal presentation at trail. Which will include visiting, possibly several law libraries and legal associations. Imagine a tort case with so many twists and turn of law. It could make anyone's head spin. Respectively, the nursing practice of the licensed practical nurse may be just as arduous as that of the paralegal. So much footwork and reading for compiling a legal action could be as exhausting as working on the patient/client unit. Take charge of it.

I have participated, as a chief nurse paralegal, on several types of personal injury, medical mal-practice and products liability cases, at the offices of personal injury attorneys', for fifteen years.

As a professionally licensed nurse, I was in charge of obtaining and reviewing medical records for trials. Including accompanying plaintiff(s) to medical offices for the plaintiff(s) and defendants, medical, surgical, physical and psychological legal examinations before trial. I took descriptive legal notes of such examination that may be included as evidence, which I witnessed at such examinations before trial. Upon reviewing medical records for application as evidence at trial, specific and detailed medically interpretive notes were conducted. The interpretation of medical and surgical terminology was converted into medical ease, for presentation to the jury. There is another type of examination before trial (EBT), where a pre-trail conference by the attorney's for both sides meet, usually with the plaintiff(s) for the hearing and pretrial questioning of the plaintiff(s) expressed details with evidence of the legal action commenced. The attorney for the plaintiff(s) will be present, in support of the plaintiff(s) defense.

Professionally licensed nurses read and document into medical and nursing records throughout their career. Not every attorney representing cases of personal injury, medical mal-practice or products liability, are well versed in such thorough and professional implementation and applications of medical or surgical terminology. I believe that no law school teaches medical/surgical as well as its scientific applications. No law school teaches on how to read and interpret medical or surgical treatments, procedures or pharmacology, for that matter. Experts in their scientific field will then be required to complete such reviews and be required to testify on such expert documents. Therefore, professionally licensed medical and nursing healthcare providers are professionally suitable for reviewing medical records and documents for the implementation as legal evidence at trials of such personal injury litigation.

As with all professions, the licensed nurse will need to be knowledgeable of appropriate laws, rules and regulations, credentialing by an accredited school or agency. Protect your license your career your family and your assets. Have an attorney for much needed consultation through out your years of professional nursing practice. A licensed practical nurse is just as vulnerable to malpractice lawsuits like medical doctors. In this litigious age of things under the microscope of society, diligent practice is the best practice. Like defensive driving on roads, the consumer of health care services is also scrutinizing how they receive health care.

First and foremost, know your scope of practice that is governed by federal, state and local laws. Also, know the policies and procedures applied to the area of practice. "Document, -document, -document!!!" Keep notes. You cannot always remember everything. Time management practice is essential, for patient/client prioritization, thus preventing chaotic confusion. After all, one never knows when the healthcare recipients' medical records may be summoned for court.

There are regulating and inspection agencies that monitor both sides of the health care delivery systems. From who is performing healthcare services, the provider of healthcare services, to who is receiving healthcare. Which may be the healthcare recipient, patient, client or institution; inclusively, providers of duly certified and licensed healthcare practitioners. They can be medical doctors, registered nurses, practical nurses, healthcare technicians or healthcare assistants. Students of healthcare educating institutions are also healthcare providers. These students are under the direct supervision of a licensed health care school and it's professional educators. Students are covered under school bonds and insurances. If a student of practical nursing is in error, inclusively, the practical nursing school instructor and the practical nursing student and the school of practical nursing may be liable for acts of commission or acts of omission: notwithstanding, the educational institution, which may be deemed as a deviation from the standards of practice. So as is legally expressed, "caveat emptor", which the legal Latin term for "buyer beware. Which may also mean "the buyer and seller of healthcare service need be conscious of such goods and services.

When a practical nursing student becomes a licensed practical nurse, duly licensed to practice as a licensed practical nurse, such licensed practical nurse is considered no longer indigenous of the laws that govern the scope of practice as a licensed nurse. This is the reason for being up to date with the standards of practice when performing professionally licensed nursing, as well as, the legal scope of practice. Unfortunately the following are not acceptable reasons or rational for incompetent delivery of care. I forgot, now I remember, oh yeah that's right, I will do right next time and tomorrow, seemingly unforgiving but not really. Mistakes can be hard lessons. Admission of mistakes may become lessons for everyone involved, hopefully, never to be repeated.

Scope of practice is a focal point of area of practice, not be confused with "this is how we do it at other areas of practice". More like a negative transference of nursing practices. That is to say, when practicing as a licensed nurse, one may learn a variety of methods and styles by which a treatment or procedure may be performed. Not all schools of practical nursing are alike. Educators of practical nurses come from different schools and clinical experiences. The educators may have different degrees and certifications. There are nursing educators who are from different backgrounds, countries and nursing exposures. Therefore, after graduating from the school of practical nursing, professional practice will have continuous changes.

New devices, medications and modes of documentation are implemented. Especially, the ever changing laws that govern and regulate the scope of practices of the professional licensed practical nurse. From observation and documentation to methods and reporting throughout the ladder of communication, the chain of command reaches higher and broader levels of professional healthcare provider and its recipients. A dynamic cliché "the customer is always right" can apply to all on the continuum of healthcare providers and healthcare recipients. Maritime and aerospace nursing are not limited to the licensed practical nurse.

Including maritime healthcare, merchant marines or mariners of the armed forces such as on ships and submarines personnel as well as amphibious vehicle personal. Maritime nurses are usually called medics or docs. Aerospace nursing at airports and launch pad areas are also military healthcare consumers, even on a privately chartered airplane, jet or helicopter. A unique set of laws will apply there as well.

While driving one day, I noticed a teleport. But I did not see anything. Not even a telephone booth. Hmmmmmmm. There were no parked cars. There were no people. The area was fenced off and the gates were closed with locks on them. Not even a house or buildings in the area. Just open road and a driveway. (S.I.)

The professionally licensed nurse can be part of traveling medical and nursing teams. Traveling from state to state, city to city, nationally or internationally. Finding your niche as a traveling professional licensed practical nurse may open the doors for professional nurse diversification. In this day and age of cell phones, satellite phones and laptops and smart pads, with hot spot communications, there is no limit to how far the licensed practical nurse can virtually go. A greater platform of professional licensed nursing practices is eminent. There will be specific healthcare voids the may be filled by the professional licensed practical nurse. Therefore, being professionally cost effective. The logistics of the economics of healthcare are shattering. Every nation and country has so much to offer for the healthcare of mankind.

Importing and exporting of health care services is as ancient Rome. The health care domain is a people's domain. If there were no persons with ills in the whole universe, there would be no need for healthcare delivery systems. Although, preventive healthcare of all, humanity and wildlife as well, will exist. Like the human body has many members so does the constellation of healthcare has a very important member and that is the professional licensed practical nurse.

Where there is a need of healthcare, there will always be a professionally licensed nurse to provide it. Aspiring to be a licensed practical nurse may begin in one continent and end up in another. Professionally licensed nurses are American licensed practical nurses. On the East coast the license practical nurse and on the West coast a licensed vocational nurse. A licensed practical nurse may have a registered nurse education, but may start their nursing practice as a licensed practical nurse. The registered nurse may be from American schools of nursing or schools of nursing in other countries. This makes the art of nursing multilingual and multicultural. Therefore, mobility in nursing as a licensed practical nurse will not be limited to where a licensed nurse went to school. Only that when in Rome do as in Rome. Another cliché' that indicates know your scope of practice the language and the population of healthcare recipients that will receive health care from you the licensed nurse.

"I raised my eyes to the heavens from where my strengths cometh, for my strengths cometh from God Who made the heavens and the earth" (Psalms 91, KJV).

Being faithful and having faith in your travels as a licensed practical nurse will always be fruitful. Changing environments will need positive degree of confidence and courage to face the ills of society and of humanity. In order to meet the healthcare needs for providing professional healthcare services to the healthcare recipient, one must be diligent. As stated in Chapter one, the health care recipient may be a private person a nursing agency a registry of licensed and certified professional medical and nursing healthcare providers, a corporation or facility, that is, a healthcare institution, school or a community. Offers and negotiations will vary from recipient to recipient. Though one should provide healthcare services for the outcome not the income.

A licensed nurse contractor/vender is a duly licensed professional nurse in the state, be it the west coast or east coast, of where the practice of professional nursing is performed. From primary medical nursing to specialty medical-surgical nursing, all health care delivery systems have a policy and procedure manual that assist with the scope of such medical and nursing practice.

The journey of the professionally licensed nurse may be taken through many paths in life. Nonetheless, enriching the professional practice of nursing throughout the healthcare continuum. A rewarding journey at that. Having experienced the mosaic of humanity and the challenges and successes of being there for every culture and way of life. Witnessing the recovery of the infirm, the weak, the broken and the lost. Just knowing that being there as best prepared as humanly possible for mankind, regardless of status, socioeconomic and traditional cultural belief. It was the most blessed experience to attain. As brief as it may have been for the client/patients served, the lasting impressions were the best take-away to be treasured. I am grateful to be in the family of healthcare providers for all humanity on all fronts.

Becoming an advanced practice licensed nurse, in the varied and diversified professional integration of professional healthcare, in recognition of the capabilities for all licensed nurses. It is well noted that when professionally educated, disciplined and trained in the vast of healthcare, professional nursing can be limitless. The greatest of all things done is knowing that selflessly giving of oneself and never asking for anything in return from the service to humanity. The comfort and dignity provided was never overwhelming. The acquisition of personal and professional maturity, through this service to mankind became a blessing. All did not come so smoothly but a blessing, nonetheless.